MedStudy

Internal Medicine
Board-Style Questions & Answers
Volume 4

Answers

Edited by

J. Thomas Cross, Jr., MD, MPH

Candace Mitchell, MD

Robert A. Hannaman, MD

MedStudy

TABLE OF CONTENTS

NOTICE: THESE BOOKS ARE MEANT TO BE USED AS AN ADJUNCT TO THE MEDSTUDY CORE CURRICULUM. THE INTERNAL MEDICINE BOARDS COVER A VAST REALM OF INFORMATION, AND BOARD SIMULATION QUESTIONS ALONE SHOULD NOT BE YOUR ONLY PREPARATION FOR THE BOARDS.

MEDSTUDY
1761 South 8th Street, Building H1
Colorado Springs, CO 80906
(800) 841-0547

GASTROENTEROLOGY

1. Answer: B

Answer: Repeat EGD.
Gastric ulcers have malignant potential, and follow-up endoscopy to confirm healing of the ulcer(s) after treatment is necessary to exclude malignancy. Any unhealed ulcers should be biopsied (multiple biopsies are essential to increase yield). Since she is better symptomatically it is not appropriate to increase her omeprazole or change her medication regimen to antacids. Based on this clinical scenario, esophageal pH monitoring and follow-up *H. pylori* titers are not indicated in this patient.

Board Testing Point: Manage and follow up gastric ulcers.

2. Answer: B

Answer: Hepatitis A and B vaccines.
Hepatitis B vaccine is a safe, effective vaccine (90% immunity in healthy patients; less if older, obese, smokers, chronic disease regarding liver/renal/DM, HIV). Adults at risk should receive 3 injections at 0, 1, and 6 months. Indications for the hepatitis B vaccine include: patients at risk from sexual exposure (multiple partners, homosexual men), health care workers, IV drug users, patients with other liver disease, HIV+ patients (50-70% seroconversion), and infants born to HBsAg-positive women. Hepatitis A is an inactivated vaccine and indicated for travelers to endemic areas, homosexual men, IV drug users, patients with other liver disease, and those with occupational risk. Hepatitis A vaccine is 95% effective after 3 weeks and 99%+ after a second dose. According to the 2005 guidelines for preventative care from the U.S. Preventive Services Task Force, tuberculosis testing for healthy adults is not recommended. Pneumococcal vaccine is indicated in patients over the age of 65 and for those with chronic medical conditions or asplenism.

Board Testing Point: Identify patients at risk for hepatitis A and B and offer vaccination.

3. Answer: A

Answer: His history of alcohol use is not a contraindication to transplantation.
While current alcohol or drug use usually precludes non-emergent transplantation, a prior history of alcoholism does not. This patient's MELD (Model End Stage Liver Disease) score is 25; patients with MELD scores > 15 are considered high priority for transplantation. MELD score is calculated using a relatively simple formula that relies on three readily available objective variables: serum creatinine (Scr; mg/dL), total bilirubin (Tbil; mg/dL), and INR (international normalized ratio). Hepatorenal syndrome has not been specifically diagnosed in this patient, and would not be an absolute contraindication to transplantation, nor would be his degree of thrombocytopenia, often seen in hypersplenism/chronic liver disease. Transaminases are a poor indicator of cirrhosis; this patient's physical examination is entirely consistent with cirrhosis. Thus, he would be a reasonable candidate for OLT (orthotopic liver transplantation).

Board Testing Point: Appropriately refer a patient for liver transplantation.

4. Answer: E

Answer: Reassurance.
This patient's clinical presentation is most consistent with Gilbert syndrome, a benign cause of hyperbilirubinemia. Approximately 9% of the population is homozygous for the disorder, diagnosed after some physiologic stressor causes increases in serum bilirubin to levels high enough to warrant laboratory evaluation. The lack of known exposures, travel, drug use, and alcohol use, as well as the normal exam and hepatitis serologies, make other diagnoses much less likely; thus, further invasive evaluation at this time is not warranted. These patients may simply be followed clinically and informed that febrile illnesses, some medications, dehydration/starvation, and other stressors may increase the bilirubin to noticeable levels (baseline bilirubin in Gilbert's patients is usually < 3.0 mg/dL; it may rise to 6.0 mg/dL).

Board Testing Point: Correctly identify Gilbert syndrome as the etiology of jaundice in a post-operative patient.

5. Answer: B

Answer: Increased serum transferrin saturation.
This patient is presenting with pseudogout (CPPD), an arthritis known to be associated with several other conditions. In patients experiencing CPPD who are younger than 60 years, laboratories should be performed to exclude the presence of the CPPD-associated conditions (hyperparathyroidism, hemochromatosis, hypophosphatasia, and hypomagnesemia). Hypothyroidism, gout, and familial hypercalciuria are also probable associations. In this question, the answer is transferrin, requiring you to recognize the association of hemochromatosis with CPPD. Other clinical features of hemochromatosis include glucose intolerance or "bronze diabetes," liver enlargement, heart failure, hypogonadism, cardiomyopathy, and rarely, hypothyroidism. Imaging studies help confirm increased iron stored in the liver, and diagnosis is confirmed by biopsy and genetic testing.

Elevated calcitonin is seen in medullary thyroid carcinoma. HLA B-27 elevations may be seen in many disorders, including seronegative spondyloarthropathy, but this patient has no evidence of this type of arthritis. Elevations in PTH are seen in hyperparathyroidism and can be associated with CPPD, but should be associated with increased serum calcium levels (not present in the question). A positive AMA is most commonly seen in primary biliary cirrhosis.

Testing Point: Associate CPPD with hemochromatosis; order the appropriate laboratory test to diagnose hemochromatosis.

6. Answer: A

Answer: Active inflammation demonstrated on liver biopsy.
Factors associated with improved outcomes in the treatment of Hepatitis B infection include low pre-treatment levels of HBV DNA, high pre-treatment levels of serum ALT, and a short duration of infection. Active inflammation on liver biopsy is also associated with good response.

Board Testing Point: Identify factors prognostic for improvement in HBV infection undergoing interferon treatment.

7. Answer: B

Answer: Colonoscopy.
Clostridium septicum may cause gas gangrene, especially in susceptible individuals, and this patient's clinical presentation is entirely consistent with a *C. septicum* hematogenous complicated soft tissue infection. The most common underlying disorders in patients with *Clostridium septicum* myonecrosis are malignancy (especially colon cancer), neutropenia, and other disorders resulting in alteration in the normal GI mucosal barrier. Another organism that requires colonoscopy when found in the blood is *Streptococcus bovis*: bacteremia with this organism is also associated with underlying GI malignancy. However, *S. bovis* does not cause myonecrosis. This patient's family history, microcytic anemia, recent constipation, and weight loss all suggest an underlying disorder of the GI tract, namely colon cancer. *Clostridium septicum* does not commonly cause endocarditis. Patients with HIV may be at increased risk of *Clostridium septicum* bacteremia; however, she is low risk for HIV infection. There is no indication for WBC chemotaxis assays or brain imaging.

Board Testing Point: Recognize myonecrosis based on clinical presentation; interpret hematologic tests of anemia and associate *C. septicum* bacteremia and myonecrosis with underlying GI malignancy.

8. Answer: D

Answer: Patient's age is younger than 40 years old.
Hepatitis C is subdivided into several serotypes. Type I is the most common serotype in the United States, but unfortunately it is also associated with the lowest response rate to treatment. Other risk factors for a poor response include increased HCV RNA levels and longer duration of infection. Age younger than 45 years has been associated with an improved response rate.

Board Testing Point: Identify prognostic factors involved in HCV treatment with PEG interferon.

9. Answer: D

Answer: Colonic mucosal subepithelial collagen deposition.
This patient's clinical presentation and laboratory testing are consistent with microscopic (collagenous) colitis. The pathogenesis of microscopic colitis is unknown, but may present as collagenous colitis (pathologically identified by collagen deposition) or lymphocytic colitis. Women are much more commonly affected than men, and the disease usually presents in middle age. NSAIDs have been implicated in the pathogenesis of microscopic colitis, which usually presents with chronic watery diarrhea without blood, and no systemic signs (fever/weight loss). Arthralgias may occur. The symptoms may subside spontaneously. Routine laboratory testing is usually unrevealing, but stool markers such as eosinophil protein X, tryptase, and myeloperoxidase may be present.

Crypt architecture disruption and abscesses, hallmarks of inflammatory bowel disease, are not present. The presentation is not consistent with amebiasis or Whipple disease. Patients with celiac sprue are more likely to show symptoms, signs, and laboratory abnormalities of malabsorption.

Board Testing Point: Differentiate microscopic colitis from other causes of chronic diarrhea.

10. Answer: A

Answer: Multifocal stricturing and dilation of intrahepatic bile ducts on cholangiography.
These findings are diagnostic for primary sclerosing cholangitis (PSC), and 90% of patients with PSC have ulcerative colitis (alternately, 5% of UC patients have PSC). These patients are usually asymptomatic and present with elevated liver biochemical tests (mainly alkaline phosphatase). AMA (antimitochondrial antibody) is positive in primary biliary cirrhosis, and usually negative in PSC. Acute viral hepatitis often shows a less obstructed picture: higher liver enzymes and less alkaline phosphatase elevation. This patient has no findings suggestive of bone-associated alkaline phosphatase elevations. Hepatocellular carcinoma may cause elevations of alkaline phosphatase; however, this patient has no risk factors for HCC or history of cirrhosis.

Board Testing Point: Identify extraintestinal manifestations of inflammatory bowel disease, including PSC.

11. Answer: D

Answer: Ciprofloxacin + loperamide.
This individual has traveler's diarrhea (TD), an entity that has been well studied and is known to respond to antibiotics. Traveler's diarrhea is the most common illness affecting travelers and presents within the first week of travel with watery diarrhea and abdominal cramping. Occasional associated symptoms include nausea, vomiting, bloating and fever. Several etiologies are responsible for cases of TD, including multiple viruses and enterotoxigenic *E. coli* (ETEC). Avoidance of contaminated foods and practicing good hand hygiene are the most effective ways to avoid TD. In most patients, TD is a self-limited, mild illness that resolves in two or three days. In patients who have more than 3 stools per 8-hour period with associated nausea, vomiting, cramping, fever or blood in the stools, the Centers for Disease Control recommends treatment with antimicrobials for a 3-5 day course. Treatment with fluoroquinolones is recommended due to high rates of *E. coli* resistance to amoxicillin and trimethoprim/sulfamethoxazole. Bismuth subsalicylate is another option for treatment, but several doses are required, and the liquid formulation stains the mucosa. If diarrhea persists during treatment, travelers should see a physician for further testing.

While antimicrobial prophylaxis is not recommended by the CDC, many travelers fill antibiotic prescriptions prior to travel and take the medication with them, using it only if they develop diarrhea. Antimotility agents (loperamide) will shorten the course of symptoms without worsening the disease but should never be used in patients with bloody diarrhea or fever as they delay clearance of the organisms and may worsen disease (according to CDC recommendations).

Board Testing Point: Identify the most common etiology of diarrhea in a traveler; determine antimicrobials are necessary and prescribe the appropriate antibiotic.

12. Answer: B

Answer: Esophagogastroduodenoscopy (EGD).
With the new onset of symptoms, advanced age, and weight loss, one is suspicious that this is pseudoachalasia (or "secondary achalasia"), clinically the same as achalasia but caused by a malignancy. Usually the malignancy is at the gastroesophageal junction. The x-ray and manometric findings may be the same as classical achalasia. However, in this case, this patient definitely needs an EGD to look for any suspicious mass. Esophageal motility is helpful in confirming the diagnosis of achalasia, but of less importance in this specific patient. One should definitely confirm the diagnosis before proceeding with treatment options like Botox or surgery. Empiric medical therapy is not indicated until you have confirmed your diagnosis.

Board Testing Point: Identify symptoms of achalasia and order the appropriate studies to evaluate achalasia in an elderly person with weight loss.

13. Answer: E

Answer: Reassurance.
The radiograph demonstrates the classic corkscrew esophagus of esophageal spasm. This is not a serious condition, and the first-line therapy should be simple reassurance. The patient should be told to avoid cold liquids, if possible. There is no need for further tests. The EGD has a very low yield in diagnosis of atypical chest pain with these specific features. There are occasional cases of esophageal spasm that are due to acid reflux. If this problem persists, then one can consider treating the reflux angle. Likewise, tricyclic antidepressants and anxiolytic agents may be helpful later on. Calcium channel antagonists, although reported in some studies years ago as being successful, are rarely helpful in actual clinical settings.

Board Testing Point: Identify the "classic corkscrew esophagus" on a radiograph.

14. Answer: A

Answer: Gastrografin swallow.
This is an example of a post-EGD esophageal perforation. This can be induced by severe vomiting, as in Boerhaave syndrome. However, most cases are after instrumentation. Suspect esophageal perforation in any patient who experiences chest or back pain after a procedure. Mackler's classic triad = vomiting, lower thoracic pain, and subcutaneous emphysema; these symptoms in a post-procedure environment can be quickly diagnosed via contrast esophagogram; but oftentimes, patients do not present with the classic triad. Esophageal perforation is an important complication that requires a timely diagnosis. Treatment is often surgical repair with chest tube drainage of any fluid collection. EGD should specifically be avoided in this situation. When this diagnosis is suspected, the contrast esophagogram offers a less expensive alternative to CT for diagnosis.

Board Testing Point: Recognize and treat a patient with symptoms of possible esophageal perforation.

15. Answer: B

Answer: EGD in 2-3 years with biopsies of the Barrett esophagus.
This patient, after successful fundoplication, still has the slight cancer risk over time, as does every other patient with Barrett esophagus. The Barrett's is not affected by surgery; it does not resolve after surgery, and there's no evidence that the cancer risk is changed. Therefore, the patient still should be in a surveillance or screening program. There is no reason to do the barium swallow now to assess dysphagia since this symptom has resolved.

Pearls for Barrett's follow-up:
- Low-grade dysplasia: repeat EGD in 3 to 6 mo.
- High-grade dysplasia: consider surgery
- No dysplasia: screening program with EGD every 2-3 years

Board Testing Point: Prescribe an appropriate screening regimen for a patient with Barrett esophagus.

16. Answer: D

Answer: *H. pylori* **ELISA with treatment if positive.**
According to the 2005 American College of Gastroenterology practice guidelines for the management of dyspepsia, "dyspepsia" is defined as having "chronic or recurrent pain or discomfort centered in the upper abdomen." Any patient having "predominant or frequent" heartburn or acid regurgitation should be considered to have gastroesophageal reflux disease until proven otherwise. Therefore, this young male patient should be diagnosed with dyspepsia, according to his symptoms. Patients with dyspepsia who are older than 55 years or complain of worrisome symptoms (bleeding, anemia, early satiety, weight loss, dysphagia or odynophagia, vomiting) or have a family history of GI cancer, previous personal GI malignancy, previous personal peptic ulcer disease or an examination revealing lymphadenopathy or an abdominal mass should undergo EGD.

Dyspeptic patients without worrisome symptoms can be managed with one of two ways:
1) test and treat for *H. pylori* using a non-invasive test; initiate a trial of acid suppression for 4-8 weeks if symptoms continue or if the *H. pylori test* is negative
2) prescribe an empiric trial of acid suppression with a proton pump inhibitor for 4-8 weeks

The test and treat option is typically employed in patient populations with a high pre-test probability for infection with *H. pylori*--i.e., those patients from populations where prevalence of *H. pylori* is moderate to high (> 10%).

Because of much discrepancy about testing versus empirically treating *H. pylori* in the GI community, you are unlikely to be given this sort of question with answers requiring you to pick between blocking acid secretion and testing for *H. pylori*.

Board Testing Point: Recognize the risk factors, symptoms, and role of *H. pylori* testing in the evaluation of dyspepsia.

17. Answer: E

Answer: Abdominal CT scan, EUS, and octreotide scintigraphy.
This is a likely case of Zollinger-Ellison syndrome with MEN type I (Wermer syndrome). Recall MEN type 1 is an autosomal dominant condition consisting of parathyroid tumors, pancreatic islet cell tumors and pituitary hyperplasia or tumors. This patient's family history of stones, her elevated calcium level and her ulcer formation is concerning for the presence of the syndrome. It's important now to try to localize the tumor(s). The primary tumor is the gastrinoma, although often the evaluation is negative. These tumors can be quite small and evade diagnosis. The CT scan, EUS, and octreotide scan are all reasonable tests that should be done to try and localize the gastric tumor. When the tumor is associated with MEN I, it may be multifocal and not be amenable to surgery. This patient should also be evaluated for parathyroid surgery if the PTH level is increased and truly responsible for the hypercalcemia. In this case, the calcium could be elevated because of the significant dehydration.

Board Testing Point: Construct a diagnosis of MEN type 1 based on clinical history, and order the appropriate evaluation for a gastrinoma.

18. Answer: B

Answer: Metoclopramide 10 mg before each meal and at bedtime.
This patient with diabetic gastroparesis may benefit from metoclopramide. This is the most effective medicine currently available for gastroparesis, but its long-term use is limited by some of the side effects. A high-fiber diet should specifically be avoided in these patients, because it may cause difficulty in emptying out the stomach. A

liquid diet is sometimes helpful if the patient is very symptomatic. Erythromycin can stimulate stomach peristaltic contractions almost immediately, but it has not been shown to be an effective medicine for long-term use in gastroparesis. Lansoprazole may be helpful as an adjunctive therapy to help heal the esophagitis, but promoting gastric emptying is more effective treatment.

Board Testing Point: Diagnose gastroparesis in a diabetic based on history and prescribe the appropriate pharmacotherapy.

19. Answer: B

Answer: Mesalamine suppositories bid.
This patient has ulcerative proctitis. Topical therapy, as in a mesalamine suppository, will provide the fastest relief of symptoms. He may require an oral agent later for maintenance therapy, but treatment typically advances in a step-wise approach, becoming more intensive when less invasive strategies fail. Prednisone or azathioprine would not be prescribed without first trying agents with fewer side effects. Giardiasis does not cause proctitis.

Board Testing Point: Diagnose ulcerative colitis based on history and biopsy results; prescribe a regimen for treatment using a step-wise approach.

20. Answer: D

Answer: Prescribe empiric metronidazole.
The history suggests this patient acquired giardiasis by drinking contaminated water from mountain streams. Empiric therapy can be initiated with metronidazole because of the presence of the epidemiologic clues and the clinical presentation. Giardiasis is not associated with fecal leukocytes or peripheral eosinophilia. Here is a cute picture of the critter in case you have to identify it on the Board exam:

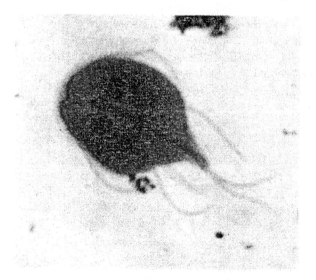

Board Testing Point: Recommend appropriate treatment for giardiasis after recognizing the epidemiologic and clinical findings of the infection.

21. Answer: C

Answer: EGD and sigmoidoscopy.
This patient is at risk for both rectal and duodenal polyps, and only this choice will evaluate the other "at risk areas" completely. He had his colon removed, but there was a segment of rectum left from the surgery. Therefore, in that very distal segment, there may be recurrent polyps that need to be surveyed. The exact intervals at which these tests should be done afterward is unknown and depends on what is found at the time of the procedures. Any rectal polyps should be removed at the time of sigmoidoscopy.

Board Testing Point: Recommend appropriate follow-up for a patient with a family history of familial polyposis.

22. Answer: B

Answer: 1 year.
After a simple polyp resection of a small adenoma, an interval of 5 years would be very reasonable. But in this case, there are 2 very large polyps, one with villous histology. Villous histology is the specific type of histology with the highest risk of having cancer and indicates a need for closer surveillance. One would not need to repeat an exam at 6 months unless there is any suspicion that all the polyp tissue had not been removed.

Board Testing Point: Identify the appropriate interval for follow-up for various types and sizes of colonic adenomas.

23. Answer: A

Answer: Acute pancreatitis.
This patient most likely has pancreatitis secondary to hypertriglyceridemia. When pancreatitis is due to hypertriglyceridemia, the amylase is often inappropriately normal. If the lipase level was ordered right now, it would be elevated and help confirm the diagnosis of pancreatitis. A perforated ulcer could certainly cause severe pain, as would cholecystitis, but these diagnoses are less likely in this setting of very high triglycerides. The perforated ulcer could be excluded with a simple upright radiograph of the abdomen. Small bowel obstruction should cause a cramping intermittent pain rather than a constant pain. Cholecystitis and gastroesophageal reflux would not have these symptoms.

Board Testing Point: Diagnose pancreatitis due to hypertriglyceridemia based on clinical history and laboratory features.

24. Answer: A

Answer: Norfloxacin.
This patient is at risk for spontaneous bacterial peritonitis, and he needs antibiotic prophylaxis to prevent this complication. Any patient with a large amount of ascites and a GI bleed is at risk. Giving lactulose is not a bad idea, and it would definitely be given if there was history of encephalopathy, but it is not as important as the norfloxacin prophylaxis. Treatment for HCV and albumin are not indicated at this time.

Board Testing Point: Recognize the potential danger of spontaneous bacterial peritonitis in a patient with large esophageal varices and ascites, and prescribe appropriate antibiotic prophylaxis.

25. Answer: D

Answer: *Staphylococcus aureus* food poisoning.
Staph aureus food poisoning is due to ingestion of a pre-formed toxin. The typical incubation period is 4 hours after eating the offending food. *Staphylococcus aureus* toxin typically resides in food that is left out for prolonged periods of time, such as in buffet settings. The symptoms are typical with vomiting followed by diarrhea. Antibiotics are ineffective in this setting because there is no active infection here. The toxin is causing the symptoms. Norovirus is the agent responsible for large outbreaks of "cruise ship diarrhea," but is rarely seen in isolated cases of vomiting and diarrhea, especially those cases implicating "buffets" or picnics. *Vibrio vulnificus* is associated with ingestion of raw seafood and sepsis with severe skin lesions. Enterohemorrhagic *E. coli* is associated with bloody diarrhea and poorly cooked hamburger.

Board Testing Point: Determine the etiology of vomiting and diarrhea on a cruise ship, utilizing clinical features and epidemiologic information.

26. Answer: A

Answer: Gallbladder ultrasound.
This patient most likely is suffering from biliary colic as a result of depletion of bile salts and cholesterol gall stone formation after ingesting a very high-fat meal. Development of cholesterol gall stones is a potential complication of severe ileal disease or resection related to Crohn's. Other complications include calcium oxalate kidney stones, B-12 deficiency, hypocalcemia (vitamin D malabsorption), and bile acid-induced diarrhea (less than 100 cm, cholestyramine). Know these potential complications. Abdominal CT requires exposure to radiation, and the diagnosis can be made with ultrasound. With these symptoms, EGD and upper GI series will not add much new information.

Board Testing Point: Identify gallstones as a complication of severe ileal disease or resection.

27. Answer: D

Answer: Encourage reduction in alcohol consumption.
Alcoholic fatty liver infiltrates can resemble those arising from non-alcoholic fatty liver disease (NAFLD) and non-alcoholic steatohepatitis (NASH). These conditions occasionally progress to further hepatic damage and cirrhosis but, overall, they tend to improve if the offending condition is alleviated. Weight loss, alcohol reduction and control of diabetes are fundamental interventions. With no evidence of liver dysfunction combined with his history of "social" alcohol consumption, the initial approach is to reduce alcohol use. Cholesterol levels are not directly tied to these deposits, and neither a statin nor a cholesterol diet will directly improve the condition. Weight loss may help, but a high carbohydrate diet without calorie control is unlikely to accomplish weight reduction. Liver biopsy and expensive studies for other liver pathology are not justified solely on the ultrasound findings, particularly in light of the normal laboratory findings.

Board Testing Point: Encourage lifestyle modification in a case of fatty liver.

28. Answer: B

Answer: A lithium battery.
Psychiatric patients have been noted to ingest a wide variety of unusual objects, and the gastrointestinal tract demonstrates a remarkable capacity to commonly pass these items. Foreign bodies that become lodged in the esophagus present a higher risk and can result in airway compromise. All of the above items may require removal if they lodge in the esophagus. Ingestion of a battery, however, is exceptionally dangerous due to the erosive chemical injury that batteries cause to the GI mucosa. Due to this risk, ingested batteries found in the esophagus are routinely removed by endoscopic or surgical procedures without delay. In general, once the ingested item has reached the jejunum, it is much more likely to pass through the GI tract without intervention. At that point, unless the foreign body causes an obstruction to the bowel or becomes lodged, it is generally observed conservatively.

Board Testing Point: Manage a patient with battery ingestion.

29. Answer: E

Answer: Reassure and offer continued follow-up.
Non-alcoholic fatty liver disease is occasionally noted on abdominal CT, MRI, or ultrasound. It is often related to diabetes mellitus, obesity, and prolonged parenteral nutrition. The most common outcome is resolution when the offending condition is improved. Some patients, however, progress to more severe liver involvement. Risk for this progression includes diabetes mellitus, obesity and an AST/ALT ratio greater than 1 (the patient in the question has none of these risk factors). Age greater than 45 years also has an increased risk, and age less than 45 is therefore associated with a better prognosis. This patient will require long-term continuity to watch for progression of disease.

Board Testing Point: Synthesize a management strategy for fatty liver based on risk factors for progression.

30. Answer: B

Answer: Schatzki ring.
The key points in this scenario are the non-painful, non-progressive dysphagia to solids but not liquids. Diffuse esophageal spasm is typically very painful (nut cracker esophagus) and involves both liquids and solids. Likewise, achalasia usually affects both liquids and solids. Barrett esophagus is related to damage to the distal esophagus and is commonly, but not always related to heartburn symptoms. It is pre-malignant and can lead to neoplastic growths that increase over time. The non-progressive nature of this patient's complaint makes this option less likely. A Schatzki ring is a lesion of the esophagus that does not usually progress and is not frequently associated with painful dysphagia. The size of the ring will determine the size of swallowed bolus that can pass. The frequency of a meat bolus resulting in symptoms has led this condition to also be referred to as "steak house dysphagia." Celiac sprue would not cause isolated esophageal symptoms.

Board Testing Point: Diagnose Schatzki ring.

31. Answer: D

Answer: Celiac disease.
She has the classic triad of dermatitis, anorexia, and abdominal distension. This triad does not fit any of the other choices listed. Celiac disease is an increasingly recognized disease process, and her history fits the disease well. Diagnosis can be confirmed with antiendomysial antibodies. Small bowel biopsy can also be done, but this

procedure is controversial as to whether it is necessary. Treatment is a gluten-free diet. Dermatitis herpetiformis is sometimes associated with celiac disease.

Board Testing Point: Interpret nebulous clinical findings in light of a high index of suspicion for celiac disease and associate celiac disease with dermatitis herpetiformis.

---

32. Answer: C

Answer: Hepatitis D infection.
He may have coinfection with hepatitis B and D or a superinfection with just hepatitis D. Remember that for hepatitis D to occur, the patient must have circulating hepatitis B surface antigen (HBsAg). He had hepatitis A in the past and is now immune. He is infectious for hepatitis B since his surface antigen is positive, but we cannot say if he is a chronic carrier based on the information presented; this requires follow-up after six months to assess whether the patient has developed antibodies against the surface antigen and effectively "cleared" the virus. His anti-HDV IgG is negative and indicates he has not yet recovered from his hepatitis D infection.

Board Testing Point: Interpret hepatitis serological testing in the setting of jaundice.

---

33. Answer: E

Answer: Supportive care.
Doxycycline is one of the most common etiologies of pill esophagitis. It typically presents when patients take doxycycline at bedtime with a small amount of liquid. It can cause severe odynophagia, leading to severe anorexia with volume depletion. This entity can be diagnosed based on clinical history. If the patient fails to improve after a few days of supportive care, EGD should be considered. Proton pump inhibitors and hyoscyamine do not improve pill esophagitis.

Board Testing Point: Recognize doxycycline as a common cause of pill esophagitis.

---

34. Answer: C

Answer: Acute hepatitis A infection and remote hepatitis B infection.
She has IgM antibody to hepatitis A virus; by definition, she has acute hepatitis A. IgG will not occur until a little later in the infection. For hepatitis B, she has "core" antibody, which indicates she has had infection at some point with hepatitis B, and since the antibody is IgG, the infection is not recent. She also has antibody to surface antigen, which means that she has "cleared the infection," and she no longer has hepatitis B surface antigen. She has never had hepatitis D infection, nor will she be able to have hepatitis D in the future; because with hepatitis D infection, you must have hepatitis B surface antigen to become infected.

Board Testing Point: Interpret hepatitis serology in a jaundiced injection drug abuser.

---

35. Answer: E

Answer: Frequent nocturnal symptoms.
All of the other symptoms are common in irritable bowel syndrome. Nocturnal symptoms are very uncommon and should suggest another diagnosis.

Board Testing Point: Identify nocturnal symptoms of diarrhea and abdominal pain as concerning for diagnoses other than irritable bowel syndrome.

36. Answer: A

Answer: Splenectomy.
Varices restricted to portions of the stomach in the absence of esophageal varices are consistent with splenic vein thrombosis. Thrombosis of the splenic vein is also associated with splenomegaly and normal hepatic function tests. The varices are not secondary to increased pressure in the hepatic portal system, and bypass procedures, such as portocaval bypass shunts or TIPS procedures, have no role in treatment. Octreotide and variceal sclerosis may abate acute bleeding but do not address the long-term cause, and bleeding can be expected to recur. The established treatment for this condition is splenectomy. Splenic vein thrombosis is often associated with pathology of the pancreas, including pancreatic masses and chronic pancreatitis.

Board Testing Point: Recognize the clinical presentation of splenic vein thrombosis.

37. Answer: C

Answer: Chest radiograph.
This patient's presentation is consistent with right lower-lobe pneumonia. The patient is febrile with tachypnea. The breaths are shallow with decreased entry into the bases. Cough and auscultatory findings are not always present in early stages of pneumonia, and irritation of the diaphragm may cause pain referral to the abdomen. A soft abdomen, normal bowel sounds, and lack of rebound lead away from a primary abdominal source of disease. Normal liver function tests, normal liver size, and no tenderness to palpation lead away from hepatic or gall bladder involvement. Normal urinalysis and lack of dysuria are not suggestive of a urinary tract infection.

Board Testing Point: Consider a diagnosis of pneumonia when it presents as abdominal pain.

38. Answer: D

Answer: Peptic stricture.
This man has had symptoms for over 2 years with slow, gradual progression. This is consistent with peptic stricture. Any patient with dysphagia for solids, but not liquids, should be suspected of having anatomic obstruction. There are 3 main causes of anatomic obstruction:
1) In younger patients, it is usually due to a Schatzki ring (lower esophageal ring). They are common and occur in 1/7 but are usually symptomatic only when the lumen has become < 13 mm diameter.
2) In older patients, it usually is carcinoma, particularly if the dysphagia is rapid in onset (over a few months) and accompanied by anorexia and weight loss. Squamous cell carcinoma of the esophagus is associated with smoking, alcohol, achalasia, and lye ingestion. Adenocarcinoma of the esophagus would be suspected if the patient had a history of GERD or Barrett esophagus.
3) Peptic stricture is the 3rd most common cause of anatomic obstruction and, again, it occurs gradually without other symptoms such as weight loss or anorexia.

Board Testing Point: Recognize anatomic causes of dysphagia and, by using the patient's symptoms, determine which etiology is most likely.

39. Answer: B

Answer: Diffuse esophageal spasm.
Dysphagia for both solids and liquids suggest an esophageal motor disorder. These include achalasia, diffuse esophageal spasm, and scleroderma involving the esophagus. Peptic stricture and Schatzki ring are anatomic obstructions, not motor disorders. Because the patient's symptoms are initiated by cold liquids, this suggests diffuse esophageal spasm. There is no good therapy for diffuse esophageal spasm, but usually attempted are calcium channel blockers, muscle relaxers, and nitrates.

Board Testing Point: Recognize the findings of diffuse esophageal spasm and be able to differentiate it from other motor disorders, such as achalasia and scleroderma.

40. Answer: D

Answer: 24-hours ambulatory esophageal pH probe.
Nonallergic asthma with nocturnal episodes may be a manifestation of GERD. The best diagnostic study for determining GERD is ambulatory esophageal pH monitoring. It would be very convincing evidence if you could document an episode of GE reflux with the onset of symptoms. Microaspiration of acidic material in the esophagus may not be necessary to produce bronchospasm; in fact, just the lowering of the pH in the esophagus alone can be sufficient to cause bronchospasm.

The upper endoscopy is not sensitive in picking up GERD since only about 2% of patients with GERD will have evidence of esophagitis. Barium swallow also has a very low sensitivity. Spirometry would not be useful since we know she already has bronchospasm, and a lung CT would provide no useful information.

Board Testing Point: Recognize that intermittent nocturnal wheezing without daytime symptoms may be a sign of GE reflux disease.

41. Answer: D

Answer: Urine for 5-HIAA.
She likely has carcinoid syndrome and in fact probably has carcinoid with a secondary niacin deficiency. The niacin deficiency causes the 3 Ds: dementia, dermatitis, and diarrhea. The carcinoid itself causes dramatic vasoactive mediator symptoms such as paroxysmal flushing, explosive diarrhea, and hypotension. Urine for 5-HIAA is a useful test and, if it is >25 mg/d, it is diagnostic for carcinoid. Lower levels (9-25 mg/d) could be carcinoid, nontropical sprue, or acute intestinal obstruction. None of the other choices will help you make the diagnosis of carcinoid syndrome.

Board Testing Point: Recognize the findings of carcinoid syndrome and its association with niacin deficiency.

42. Answer: B

Answer: Low-fat diet and medium-chain triglyceride supplements.
In this instance, where > 100 cm of distal ileum has been removed, steatorrhea will occur. This is due to decreased bile acids. This condition is best treated with low-fat diet and supplemental medium-chained triglycerides. When less than 100 cm of distal ileum is removed, patients with diarrhea usually have bile-induced diarrhea, which is best treated with cholestyramine. She has no evidence of bacterial overgrowth (no need for metronidazole) and no evidence of pancreatic insufficiency.

Board Testing Point: Recognize the findings of iatrogenic steatorrhea.

43. Answer: E

Answer: Mesalamine suppositories should be initiated now.
He has ulcerative proctitis. The duration of 3 months generally excludes a bacterial colitis. It is possible for a patient with proctitis to have extension of the disease process to involve the entire colon; however this is not common and occurs in < 20%. Most patients will usually have recurring disease in the distal segment. Ulcerative proctitis is not associated with an increased risk of cancer and does not require systemic corticosteroids usually for therapy. Many treatments are appropriate, including mesalamine suppositories or oral sulfasalazine, but the fastest relief would be with the mesalamine suppositories.

Board Testing Point: Recognize the findings of ulcerative proctitis.

44. Answer: C

Answer: Colonoscopy as soon as can be scheduled.
Her father died at a young age from colon cancer. Hereditary GI disease must be ruled out, including familial colonic polyposis and Gardner syndrome. Gardner syndrome is characterized by multiple colonic adenomas, while familial colonic polyposis has hundreds of colonic adenomas. Risk of cancer in each of these is 100% if not treated with proctocolectomy. Colonoscopy is the procedure of choice.

CT scan of the abdomen is not likely to be helpful and will not give you tissue if you find an abnormal finding. EGD is not indicated and neither is gallium scan. For most people with an early family history (non-syndromic or non-hereditary type) of colon cancer, it is best to start screening 10 years earlier than the time the diagnosis was made in the older family member.

Board Testing Point: Recognize that early screening is necessary in patients with family members who have been diagnosed with colon cancer at early ages.

45. Answer: E

Answer: Erythromycin 500 mg bid for 5 days.
This patient has *Campylobacter* infection. In general, antibiotics are not the cornerstone of treatment of *C. jejuni* gastroenteritis. Maintenance of proper hydration and correction of electrolyte imbalance should be the focus. Antimicrobial therapy should be used only in patients who are severely ill, elderly, pregnant, or immunocompromised. Other groups in whom antibiotic therapy is indicated include those with bloody stools (our patient), high fever, extraintestinal infection, worsening symptoms or relapses, and those with symptoms lasting longer than one week (our patient again). Erythromycin is the drug of choice for *Campylobacter* infection. This is

the only common diarrheal infection that you treat with erythromycin, so remember it because it is different! The other antibiotic choices listed are generally ineffective for *Campylobacter* infection.

Infection with *Shigella* almost always requires therapy: trimethoprim-sulfamethoxazole (if sensitive) or ciprofloxacin. With uncomplicated *Salmonella* gastroenteritis, antibiotic therapy is not indicated. If you treat *Salmonella* with antibiotics, you risk prolonging shedding, as well as increasing the risk of resistance. Remember: *Shigella* you treat; *Salmonella* you generally don't. Exceptions for the treatment of *Salmonella* are the very old, the very young, and the immunocompromised. We treat these patients with antibiotics because the risk that the *Salmonella* may disseminate or cause more extensive problems is greater than the risk of prolonged shedding.

Board Testing Point: Prescribe the appropriate antibiotic treatment when appropriate for patients with *Campylobacter jejuni.*

PULMONOLOGY

46. Answer: B

Answer: Adenosine deaminase.
Tuberculous pleural effusions are usually exudative and are characteristically high in lymphocytes: more than 50% lymphocytes in a pleural tap should prompt a search for TB as the cause of the effusion, and absence of mesothelial cells is also suggestive. Pleural cultures are less helpful because only 40% are sensitive for TB. Multiple pleural biopsies increase the yield greatly, but cultures/biopsy may delay diagnosis. Adenosine deaminase (ADA) is both sensitive and specific for pleural tuberculosis (using ADA cutoff for normal of 40 U/L; sensitivity = 99.6%, specificity = 97.1%). Abnormally low pleural glucose may be seen in infectious and rheumatoid effusions but is nonspecific. In chylothorax, triglycerides will be elevated; there are many causes including malignancy, thoracic duct obstruction, and TB. TB is the most common cause of pseudo-chylothorax, but the pleural fluid in pseudo-chylothorax will show elevated cholesterol rather than triglycerides.

Board Testing Point: Identify the best method to diagnose a tuberculous pleural effusion.

47. Answer: B

Answer: Bupropion.
Thromboangiitis obliterans has a well-recognized association with cigarette smoking, although the mechanism of the pathology is not entirely clear. Patients with this condition often have significant difficulty abstaining from tobacco products. Nicotine is felt to play a role in the pathogenesis, and nicotine products used for smoking cessation may perpetuate the process. Corticosteroids have no role in smoking cessation and have not been shown to benefit the inflammatory process of thromboangiitis obliterans. Benzodiazepines have no role in either smoking cessation or thromboangiitis obliterans. Bupropion has some efficacy in smoking cessation and is not known to directly affect the pathogenesis of thromboangiitis obliterans. It does lower seizure thresholds and should not be used in patients with known seizure disorders.

Board Testing Point: Recommend appropriate therapy for smoking cessation in a patient with Buerger disease.

48. Answer: E

Answer: Selective bronchial artery embolization.
The patient has massive hemoptysis that is likely due to an aspergillus fungus ball that has grown in a pre-existing cavity. The hemoptysis is likely to continue without some therapy. The pre-existing cavity usually means there is devitalized tissue, as well as scar tissue that can make emergency surgery risky. Bronchial artery embolization has emerged as an attractive first step to stabilize the patient until medical treatment and elective surgical resection can be accomplished. Amphotericin B alone is not effective in resolving the fungus ball, and this is not tuberculosis, so tuberculosis therapy is not indicated.

Board Testing Point: Provide effective therapy for massive hemoptysis in the setting of a fungus ball.

49. Answer: E

Answer: Patients with an acute exacerbation of COPD with hypercapnic acidosis.
Noninvasive positive pressure ventilatory (NPPV) support is best utilized in an awake, cooperative patient with hypercapnic respiratory failure. A number of studies have demonstrated improvements in mortality in this patient population, who are treated with noninvasive ventilatory support compared to invasive strategies. Those patients who are hemodynamically unstable should be intubated and managed with invasive positive pressure ventilatory support. The same is true for patients with excessive secretions, high risk for emesis, or facial deformities/injuries that prevent proper use of a face mask for NPPV.

Board Testing Point: Identify patients for whom noninvasive positive pressure ventilation is beneficial.

50. Answer: C

Answer: Add inhaled corticosteroids to short-acting beta agonists.
This patient has moderate, persistent asthma, which is bronchodilator-responsive. The National Asthma Education and Prevention Program (NAEPP) defines moderate, persistent asthma as 1) daily symptoms requiring rescue use of short-acting beta agonists, 2) exacerbations that affect activity more than once per week, and 3) FEV_1 or peak expiratory flows between 60 and 80% of predicted normal. To be considered bronchodilator-responsive, FEV_1 must improve by 12% or 200cc; this patient increased 16%, so albuterol use is appropriate. Initial treatment for moderate, persistent asthma should be inhaled corticosteroids, with beta-agonists used for "rescue." If symptoms persist, a second "controller" agent may be added, but use of long-acting beta-agonists (LABAs; e.g., salmeterol) is not recommended for monotherapy: "LABAs should not be the first medicine used to treat asthma. LABAs should be added to the asthma treatment plan only if other medicines do not control asthma, including the use of low- or medium-dose corticosteroids." *http://www.fda.gov/cder/drug/advisory/LABA.htm*

Board Testing Point: Recognize the diagnosis and treatment of bronchodilator-responsive, moderate, persistent asthma.

51. Answer: A

Answer: Post-intubation medication effect after administration of sedatives/analgesics.
Hypotension after intubation is a common occurrence and has a number of potential causes: tension pneumothorax secondary to barotrauma, auto-PEEP secondary to aggressive bagging, post-intubation medication effect, and decreased pre-load are the most common causes. Medications and the act of intubation may decrease sympathetic output in the distressed patient. Aggressive bagging can overcome the time constant of the lung and result in auto-PEEP, which is associated with an increased intrathoracic pressure, decreased venous return, and subsequently, hypotension and decreased cardiac output. Positive pressure ventilation can also decrease blood pressure in a manner similar to auto-PEEP, which also is related to the positive intrathoracic pressure effect on venous return. The other choices listed are much less likely in a patient with recent intubation.

Board Testing Point: Identify a common etiology of hypotension after intubation.

52. Answer: E

Answer: Increase the expiratory time to allow complete exhalation and avoid breath stacking.
Auto-PEEP can be corrected by increasing the expiratory time to allow complete exhalation and avoid the stacking of breaths. This can be accomplished by shortening inspiration using either decreased tidal volumes or an

increase in inspiratory flow rates. The expiratory cycle can be increased by decreasing the number of breaths. Airflow obstruction and increased airway resistance can be improved by the administration of bronchodilator medications. In the patient on assist-control ventilatory support, decreasing the triggering sensitivity of the ventilator may decrease the machine respiratory rate, but the patient may still exert efforts in an attempt to obtain a breath resulting in an increase in patient ventilator dyssynchrony.

Board Testing Point: Identify a management strategy to correct auto-PEEP.

53. Answer: D

Answer: Active bleeding diathesis in a patient with a documented lower-extremity DVT.
IVC filters are indicated for the prevention of pulmonary emboli in patients with lower extremity thrombi who are unable to undergo anticoagulation related to a bleeding diathesis, or who have a documented failure of adequate anticoagulation to prevent a subsequent PE. IVC filters will not provide protection from PE for right ventricular thrombi or upper extremity thrombi. In this setting, adequate anticoagulation with warfarin requires the INR to be 2-3; hence, this patient is not adequately anti-coagulated.

Board Testing Point: Identify indications for placement of an inferior vena caval filter.

54. Answer: D

Answer: Seizure disorder.
Tobacco exposure is a leading cause of environment-related cancers. Smoking cessation is one of the most effective interventions for reducing the incidence of malignancies. Primary care providers should be adept at assisting patients with their efforts to discontinue their tobacco exposure. Bupropion is an approved intervention that can be helpful for some patients to reduce or eliminate tobacco usage. It is known to reduce seizure threshold and should not be used in a person with a known seizure tendency. It is frequently used as an anti-depressant. It is metabolized by the liver with metabolites excreted in the urine, and caution should be exercised for use in patients with renal impairment. Cases of hypertension, some with significant blood pressure elevations, have been reported with bupropion use, but having coexistent hypertension is not a contraindication to using the drug. Migraine headaches are an infrequent side effect.

Board Testing Point: Recognize the contraindications to the use of bupropion for smoking cessation.

55. Answer: A

Answer: Worsening hypoxemia and hypercapnia.
Auto-PEEP can result in dynamic hyperinflation with subsequent increased work of breathing and dyspnea. The positive intrathoracic pressure seen in auto-PEEP decreases venous return to the right side of the heart with subsequent decrease in pre-load and cardiac output. This can result in hypotension. The PEEP effect can be unevenly distributed within the lung and produce ventilation perfusion abnormalities with resultant hypoxemia and/or hypercapnia.

Board Testing Point: Recognize the adverse consequences of auto-PEEP.

56. Answer: A

Answer: Pulmonary embolism protocol chest CT scan with leg follow-through.
The patient in this clinical scenario has a high clinical suspicion for the presence of a pulmonary embolus. Therefore, the best single initial test would be a PE protocol chest CT with leg follow-through. An ABG would not be helpful in establishing a diagnosis of PE. Similarly, a D-Dimer, if elevated in this situation, would not help establish a diagnosis of PE. However, a negative D-Dimer could be useful in eliminating the diagnosis from the differential list. Since this patient has an abnormal chest x-ray, a ventilation perfusion lung scan may not be as useful as it would be if the chest x-ray were normal. In addition, VQ lung scans are only useful if they fall in the normal or high-probability group, and these scans do not evaluate the presence of leg clots. Doppler ultrasound exams will not detect a PE, an IVC or pelvic vein clot, and may be normal in the setting of a documented pulmonary embolus.

Board Testing Point: Recommend appropriate testing in the setting of a possible pulmonary embolism.

57. Answer: C

Answer: *Pseudomonas aeruginosa, Staphylococcus aureus, Acinetobacter sp., Enterobacter sp.*
The organisms associated with late-onset ventilator-associated pneumonia (occurring after 4 days of ventilatory support) are typical ICU-acquired organisms and include *Pseudomonas aeruginosa, Staphylococcus aureus, Acinetobacter sp.*, and *Enterobacter sp.* Typically, the *Staphylococcus aureus* will be MRSA.

Board Testing Point: Recognize the organisms responsible for late-onset, ventilator-associated pneumonia.

58. Answer: A

Answer: Managing the patient in a semi-recumbent position (head at 30° of elevation).
Elevating the head of the bed at least 30° has been shown to prevent the development of ventilator-associated pneumonia. Selective digestive decontamination of the GI tract and upper airway has been shown to reduce the development of VAP, but does not improve mortality. This technique has not been advocated because of issues related to its cost, labor requirements, and potential development of resistant organisms. Routine use of prophylactic antibiotics has not been shown to be beneficial in the prevention of VAP. Continuous aspiration of subglottic secretions has been shown to reduce VAP, but there are no data for subglottic antibiotic administration. Studies have demonstrated increased VAP with more frequent changes and interruptions of the ventilator tubing.

Board Testing Point: Identify effective strategies to prevent the development of a ventilator-associated pneumonia (VAP).

59. Answer: B

Answer: Absence of elevated left heart filling pressure.
The American-European Consensus Conference definition of ARDS incorporates a statement for an at-risk situation: bilateral infiltrates visible on frontal radiograph, oxygenation abnormality manifested by a $P_aO_2/F_iO_2 < 200$, and absence of left heart failure (normal left ventricular filling pressures).

Board Testing Point: Identify criteria for the diagnosis of ARDS.

60. Answer: C

Answer: Effect of fluticasone.
There are several types of agents available for the treatment of asthma. These include both long- and short-acting beta-agonists, oral and inhaled corticosteroids, mast cell stabilizers, and antibiotics for infectious episodes. Among these, inhaled steroids (e.g., fluticasone) have been associated with vocal cord dysfunction, ranging from hoarseness to aphonia. The condition usually resolves upon withdrawal of the inhaled steroid from the treatment regimen. Independent association of aphonia with the other agents listed has not been identified.

Board Testing Point: Recognize the side effects of inhaled steroids.

61. Answer: D

Answer: D. Methotrexate is useful in steroid-resistant cases.
Treatment for sarcoidosis remains somewhat controversial since many of the cases resolve spontaneously, and long-term permanent changes are often resistant to treatment. Elevated ACE levels have been noted in many sarcoid patients, but ACE inhibitors play no role in the treatment, except they are useful in hypertension for these patients! There is limited evidence for implication of infectious etiologies in sarcoid development, but macrolide antibiotics do not result in improvement. Steroids are the principal tool of therapy, but inhaled steroids are ineffective in reducing pulmonary sarcoidosis. Methotrexate is the second-line agent for patients who do not respond to steroids.

Board Testing Point: Identify methotrexate as useful for treatment of refractory sarcoidosis.

62. Answer: D

Answer: Recently, there has been an increase in the number of virulent and resistant organisms causing CAP. This includes community-acquired methicillin-resistant *Staphylococcus aureus* (MRSA).
Typically, the causative organism for CAP is not found in more than 50% of cases. For optimum outcome, antibiotics should be administered in less than 8 hours, preferably less than 4 hours from presentation. There has been a recent increase in the number of virulent organisms in the community, which includes MRSA. There is little scientific data and controlled trial evidence to provide guidance on how long to treat CAP. Recent trials with levofloxacin find that 5 days of 750 mg was sufficient.

Board Testing Point: Recognize that more resistant organisms are responsible for CAP today.

63. Answer: A

Answer: Penicillin-resistant *Streptococcus pneumoniae*.
The risk factors for penicillin-resistant *Streptococcus pneumoniae* infection include age > 65 years, prior receipt of beta-lactam antibiotics in the past 3 months, exposure to children in daycare, multiple medical comorbidities, and residence in a nursing home. Prior receipt of the pneumococcal vaccine does not increase a patient's risk for acquiring penicillin-resistant *Streptococcus pneumoniae*.

Board Testing Point: Recognize risk factors for penicillin-resistant *Streptococcus pneumoniae*.

64. Answer: C

Answer: Pulmonary angiogram.
In the setting of a high clinical suspicion for PE and a non-diagnostic PE protocol CT with leg follow-through, the next best exam for evaluating the presence or absence of a pulmonary embolus would be to use the "gold standard," a pulmonary angiogram. A Doppler ultrasound exam of the lower extremities and arms may be helpful in finding a DVT if the leg follow-through was less than optimal. Transthoracic echocardiography has a poor ability to detect a pulmonary embolus, but a transesophageal echocardiogram may pick up a central clot. The other choices listed at this point in the evaluation are not going to add useful information.

Board Testing Point: Recommend a pulmonary angiogram when there is a high clinical suspicion of pulmonary embolism and a negative high-quality CT study.

65. Answer: E

Answer: All of the choices are correct.
This is not a true Board-style question, but was placed here to remind you of factors to consider in community acquired *Pseudomonas* infections. The Boards will expect you to be on the lookout for these during the examination. The risk factors for *Pseudomonas* as an etiologic organism in community-acquired pneumonia include the use of broad-spectrum antibiotics for greater than 7 days during the past month, administration of immunosuppressive regimens (including prednisone doses of > 10 mg/day), residence in a nursing home or chronic health care setting, malnutrition, and the presence of structural lung disease, such as bronchiectasis. While chronic dialysis is a risk factor for Gram-negative infection and health care-associated pneumonia, it is not a risk factor for *Pseudomonas* pneumonia.

Board Testing Point: Know the risk factors for *Pseudomonas* infection.

66. Answer: C

Answer: Receiving home medical care, such as infusion therapy, wound care, etc.
Health care-associated pneumonia is a relatively new designation for a form of community-acquired pneumonia that is found in patients who reside in institutional settings, have chronic health care needs, have had recent antibiotic treatment, or who were recently discharged from the hospital (hospitalized for at least 2 days within 90 days, not 120 days, as listed in one of the choices). The etiology of health care-associated pneumonia has a different microbiological spectrum compared to community-acquired pneumonia; and hence, requires a different antimicrobial treatment regimen.

Board Testing Point: Identify the criteria for health care-associated pneumonia.

67. Answer: A

Answer: Support oxygenation and maintain an oxygen saturation of 88% or greater.
The typical goals of mechanical ventilatory support are to achieve and maintain adequate oxygenation. This is defined as a saturation of greater than or equal to 88%. Care should be taken to avoid normalizing the P_aCO_2 in all patients. This is particularly true in patients who have a baseline elevated P_aCO_2 related to obstructive lung disease or OSA/CSA or in those patients who have hyperventilated to compensate for a metabolic acidosis. In both cases, undesirable pH changes will result. Recent emphasis has been placed on avoiding alveolar overdistention to minimize the potential for ventilator-induced lung injury. Maintaining the end-inspiratory plateau pressure less than or equal to 30 cm H_2O should minimize the potential for alveolar overdistention. Complete rest of the diaphragm and respiratory muscles has theoretical value in states of compromised cardiac output and oxygen delivery. Routine utilization will prolong ventilatory requirements as a result of atrophy of these muscles.

Board Testing Point: Recognize the goals of mechanical ventilatory support.

68. Answer: A

Answer: Employ a lung-protective ventilatory support strategy using a low tidal volume and nomogram-guided PEEP, since this strategy has been shown to improve survival for patients with ALI and ARDS.
The ARDS network demonstrated that the use of lung-protective, low tidal volume ventilatory support and PEEP dosed according to a nomogram improved survival compared to large tidal volume ventilatory support. This strategy maintains the end-inspiratory plateau pressure less than 30 cm H_2O to avoid alveolar overdistention (volutrauma) and provides for adequate PEEP to prevent recurrent recruitment-derecruitment (atelectatic-trauma). The use of albumin infusions, coupled with furosemide in hypoproteinemic patients with ALI/ARDS, has recently been shown in a small pilot trial to improve oxygenation and fluid balance compared to administration of furosemide and placebo, but did not significantly improve survival. Prone positioning typically results in improved oxygenation; this is in part related to getting the heart off of the left lower lobe. Inhaled nitric oxide, like prone positioning, has been shown in a number of trials to improve oxygenation early after application. However, despite this improved oxygenation seen with inhaled nitric oxide and prone positioning, there was not an improvement in survival.

Board Testing Point: Recognize that low tidal volume and nomogram-guided PEEP has improved survival in patients with ALI and ARDS.

69. Answer: D

Answer: Panic attack.
Calculation of the A-a gradient on room air determines a value of 18 mm Hg. This is a normal value, indicating no problems at the alveolar capillary unit. The most likely explanation is supratentorial hyperventilation as deduced by interpreting the blood gas.

Board Testing Point: Utilize the A-a gradient as a diagnostic tool.

70. Answer: D

Answer: Pulmonary edema.
V/Q mismatch is the most common reason for hypoxemia involving the alveolar-capillary unit (all of the other choices listed cause hypoxemia in this manner). A diffusion defect is almost never the cause of hypoxemia at rest, except in the case of pulmonary edema.

Intrapulmonary shunt physiology is the cause of hypoxemia in situations when large numbers of alveoli are totally collapsed (major atelectasis) or full of something other than air (CHF, ARDS, or lobar pneumonia).

Board Testing Point: Recognize that pulmonary edema results in hypoxemia due to diffusion defect, not an alveolar-capillary unit abnormality.

71. Answer: E

Answer: Oxygen.
The blood gases drawn on this patient show a mild metabolic acidosis and a violation of the 30-60...60-90 rule for oxyhemoglobin saturation. With a P_aO_2 greater than 60 torr, hemoglobin saturation should exceed 90%. When this does not occur, something else has displaced oxygen from the hemoglobin. The night spent in the RV during November suggests that the culprit is carbon monoxide. Interestingly, the amount of oxygen dissolved in the plasma (P_aO_2) is often normal in carbon monoxide poisoning. Treatment with supplemental oxygen will displace the carbon monoxide from the hemoglobin and return the patient to normal homeostasis.

Board Testing Point: Recognize the presentation and effective treatment of carbon monoxide poisoning.

72. Answer: C

Answer: Total Lung Capacity (TLC).
The Total Lung Capacity is an important variable for making the diagnosis of restrictive lung disease. It is calculated by measuring the residual volume (RV) and then adding the resting Vital Capacity (VC). The RV is difficult to measure accurately, and 3 methods can be used: helium dilution, nitrogen washout, or body plethysmography. Of these, the body plethysmography is the most accurate.

Board Testing Point: Identify the measurable parameters of pulmonary function testing; recognize that the TLC is a calculated value.

73. Answer: C

Answer: Perform PFTs with a flow-volume loop.
All patients deserve PFTs to document suspected asthma. A flow-volume loop will provide additional information regarding the upper airway that would help diagnose vocal cord problems or benign adenomas as alternate causes of wheezing. This appears to be exercise-induced and bronchoprovocation may not be helpful. Medications may be helpful but should be prescribed after the diagnosis is more clearly defined. This patient had a pattern consistent with a fixed upper airway obstruction likely due to prior intubation during his bout with Guillain-Barré syndrome.

Board Testing Point: Recommend the initial step in evaluation of suspected asthma.

74. Answer: A

Answer: Throat culture and tuberculosis skin testing.
The skin lesions in this patient are consistent with erythema nodosum (EN). Several conditions are associated with the development of EN. Strep infections are a leading cause and, with the findings noted on chest x-ray, tuberculosis is also a strong consideration. Sarcoidosis is a strong consideration, especially in this young adult with EN, respiratory findings, and a typical pattern on chest radiograph. The diagnosis of sarcoidosis, however, depends on clinical correlation of historical, radiographic, and histological evidence, not based on an elevation of the ACE-level or lack thereof. There is no definitive diagnostic test. Lung biopsy typically shows non-caseating granulomas, but several other processes can also produce the same clinical picture. Kveim-Siltzbach testing is no longer used secondary to difficulties obtaining standardized testing reagents. ACE levels are commonly elevated but not in a predictable or specific fashion. Biopsy of erythema nodosum does not contain tissue that clarifies the differential diagnosis.

Board Testing Point: Identify etiologies of erythema nodosum.

75. Answer: E

Answer: Mechanical ventilation.
This patient has status asthmaticus that is severe by clinical presentation. The objective measurement of PEFR using the 100-200-300 rule justifies immediate admission. Expected arterial blood gas interpretation in states of status asthmaticus is hypoxemia with respiratory alkalosis. "Normal-appearing" ABGs indicate that the patient is tiring, and the respiratory acidosis suggests that some form of positive pressure breathing support will be required. Based on his ABGs and clinical findings, only mechanical ventilation provides a good solution. He cannot ventilate on his own, and neither antibiotics nor a heliox 70/30 mask is going to alleviate this. Also more studies, such as CXR or spirometry, will not add any useful information.

Board Testing Point: Direct appropriate therapy for a patient with status asthmaticus with acidemia and respiratory acidosis.

76. Answer: D

Answer: Using low inspiratory flow rates to maintain peak inspiratory pressures less than 30 cm H_2O.
Auto-PEEP results when the time constant of the lung is violated. This typically occurs in clinical settings with increased airway resistance and/or increased airway compliance. However, auto-PEEP can occur whenever there is not enough time for complete exhalation to occur before the next breath is delivered and stacking of breaths occurs. Any condition that shortens the expiratory phase of the respiratory cycle, such as the use of low inspiratory flow rates, large tidal volumes, or increased respiratory rates will predispose to the development of auto-PEEP.

Board Testing Point: Recognize the factors that are associated with development of auto-PEEP.

77. Answer: C

Answer: Administration of corticosteroids.
All asthmatics with an attack significant enough to require ED care should receive corticosteroids. Even though systemic steroids may not begin to have a meaningful effect for 3-4 hours, they will protect against or ameliorate the late-phase reactions of asthma. In the absence of vomiting, oral systemic steroids, such as prednisone, can be

given in lieu of intravenous because of their rapid absorption and complete bioavailability. Oral steroids have been shown to be as effective as intravenous.

Board Testing Point: Identify systemic corticosteroids as necessary therapy in an acute exacerbation.

78. Answer: A

Answer: Add a long-acting beta-2 inhaler to current regimen.
Until the recent introduction of effective long-acting beta-2 inhalers, the strategy would have been to increase the inhaled corticosteroids. It is now known that the addition of a long-acting beta-2 agonist (salmeterol) is more effective than doubling the dose of steroids. Be sure you know the protocols for step-wise management: the use of theophylline, allergy testing, or oral steroids is not indicated at this juncture.

Board Testing Point: Recommend the appropriate step-wise management of asthma.

79. Answer: C

Answer: Asthma.
Creola bodies, Curschmann spirals, and Charcot-Leyden crystals are all representative of eosinophilic breakdown material and can be found in the sputum of some asthmatics. Their presence signifies an increase in the eosinophilic content of the sputum, but do not represent infection with *Aspergillus*. The brown flecks sometimes found in the sputum of patients with ABPA are actual fragments of the organism.

Board Testing Point: Know the significance of finding Charcot-Leyden crystals.

80. Answer: A

Answer: Asthma.
The 3 most common causes of chronic cough are sinusitis with post-nasal drip, gastroesophageal reflux, and cough variant asthma. Of the choices listed, only cough-variant asthma would be a likely diagnosis. None of the other choices would present in this manner.

Board Testing Point: Recognize asthma as a cause of chronic cough.

81. Answer: B

Answer: Aspergilloma.
The finding of a mass within a cavity suggests the presence of a mycetoma or "fungus ball." The cavity is typically pre-existing and subsequently colonized by *Aspergillus*. After a period of growth, the *Aspergillus hyphae* cause irritation and erosion of the cavity wall with resultant hemoptysis. Treatment is typically bronchial artery embolization rather than immediate surgery. None of the other choices would have this clinical presentation.

Board Testing Point: Recognize *Aspergillus* as a cause of aspergilloma.

82. Answer: D

Answer: Sarcoidosis.
The enlarged hilar adenopathy in a young African-American patient who is asymptomatic and feeling capable of manual labor suggests that sarcoidosis is the likely diagnosis. His review of systems being negative is not consistent with the diagnoses of lymphoma and tuberculosis. Cytomegalovirus and brucellosis do not have this clinical presentation. If necessary, bronchoscopy with transbronchial biopsies could further support the diagnosis.

Board Testing Point: Diagnose sarcoidosis based on genetic risk, history, and physical examination findings.

83. Answer: C

Answer: Lung carcinoma.
The patient's occupational history and chest radiograph findings are consistent with significant asbestos exposure. The finding of bilateral crackles is consistent with pulmonary fibrosis. Diaphragmatic pleural calcifications that are isolated can occur after exposure to asbestos. When these calcifications are found in a setting of no other lung infection or trauma, asbestos exposure should be sought in the history. Significant asbestos exposure is an independent risk factor for bronchogenic carcinoma, mesotheliomas and gastrointestinal neoplasms. The other choices listed are not at increased risk in patients with asbestos exposure.

Board Testing Point: Recognize occupational history as important in determining risk factors for lung cancer.

84. Answer: A

Answer: Coal worker's pneumoconiosis.
Coal worker's pneumoconiosis is characterized by the development of focal emphysema around acanthotic nodules. The widespread focal emphysema gives a predominantly obstructive pattern on PFTs rather than the restrictive pattern usually anticipated. Two other conditions, LAM and Histiocytosis X, also have predominantly obstructive patterns. The other choices listed are predominantly restrictive diseases.

Board Testing Point: Identify obstructive PFTs associated with coal worker's pneumoconiosis.

85. Answer: E

Answer: Treat the patient supportively with flumazenil.
Calculation of the A-a gradient on room air determines a normal value of 15 mm Hg. The normal A-a gradient interpreted in conjunction with the hypercapnia identifies the cause of hypoxemia as hypoventilation. There is no evidence that the alveolar-capillary unit has been affected, as would be the case with the immediate injury of aspiration. The cause of hypoxemia is respiratory depression from substance ingestion only and does not require interventions to address metabolic acidosis (bicarbonate infusion).

Board Testing Point: Utilize the A-a gradient as a diagnostic tool.

86. Answer: C

Answer: Pulmonary neoplasm.
Of the choices given, only neoplasm causes large accumulations of pleural fluid that would occupy 50% of the thorax. The other choices could cause pleural effusions but of much smaller volumes.

Board Testing Point: Recognize that lung cancer causes significant large volume pleural effusions.

87. Answer: E

Answer: Emphysema.
The two most common pulmonary causes of a decreased DLCO are interstitial lung disease (ILD) and emphysema. ILD typically has a restrictive pattern with a preserved FEV1/FVC ratio. This patient has obstructive lung disease as evident in his PFTs and radiograph; emphysema is the most likely cause. The DLCO is not significantly decreased in the other obstructive lung diseases listed. It is often helpful in distinguishing chronic bronchitis from emphysema, although considerable overlap can be present.

Board Testing Point: Recognize the clinical, laboratory, and x-ray findings of emphysema.

88. Answer: C

Answer: Infertility.
Most males with cystic fibrosis (95%) are infertile due to defects in sperm transport and blockage of the spermatic ducts. However, close to 80% of females remain fertile, and maternal and fetal outcomes are generally favorable if the prepregnancy FEV1 exceeds 50% to 60% of the predicted value. All of the other choices are equally likely in men or women with cystic fibrosis.

Board Testing Point: Recognize that cystic fibrosis commonly causes infertility in males but not females.

89. Answer: A

Answer: Radiographic evidence of lower lobe bullae.
Alpha-1 antitrypsin deficiency can account for 1-3% of emphysema. It usually occurs in smokers at an early age, tends to run in families, and causes lower lobe bullae rather than upper lobe bullae. Because alpha-1 antitrypsin is produced in the liver and cannot be released, many patients will develop otherwise unexplained hepatic disease.

Board Testing Point: Recognize the factors associated with emphysema that are due to alpha-1 antitrypsin deficiency.

90. Answer: A

Answer: Occupational exposure to cadmium fumes.
Up to 15% of fixed obstructive disease has been attributed to factors other than cigarette smoking. High dust exposures, as well as cadmium fumes, have been associated with COPD. Other potential etiologies include: alpha-1-antitrypsin deficiency, severe and poorly controlled childhood asthma, and coal worker's pneumonoconiosis. Airway remodeling in poorly controlled asthma may cause fixed obstructive disease in

approximately 16% of such patients. None of the other choices have been associated with fixed obstructive lung disease.

Board Testing Point: Identify risk factors associated with fixed obstructive lung disease.

---

91. Answer: E

Answer: Continuous low-flow oxygen therapy for chronic hypoxemia.
Therapy for COPD is palliative and directed at improving the quality of life. The only intervention that prolongs survival is low-flow oxygen therapy for chronic hypoxemia. Oxygen must be used continuously (> 18 h/d), and the survival benefit is not apparent until after 36 months of use.

Board Testing Point: Identify oxygen therapy as the only intervention that improves survival in patients with COPD.

---

92. Answer: D

Answer: Anticholinergic inhaled therapy as an adjunct to beta-agonist therapy.
Mucolytic agents, oral sedation, and chest physiotherapy are contraindicated in most asthmatics, whose condition will be worsened with their use. Anticholinergic therapy is complementary to beta-agonist use. Antibiotic therapy is usually not indicated in asthma attacks since the major infectious trigger is viral infection or allergies. Likewise, intravenous aminophylline and intravenous magnesium usually have little to add to properly administered beta-agonists.

Board Testing Point: Recommend a treatment strategy for acute exacerbation of asthma.

---

93. Answer: E

Answer: Begin a trial of BiPAP (Bilevel Positive Airway Pressure) by mask.
Given the patient's degree of hypercarbia, the greatest concern should be directed toward adequate ventilation. Noninvasive ventilation with continuous positive pressure delivery (BiPAP) has been successful in reducing the number of actual endotracheal intubations that are required in exacerbations of COPD, thus lessening both morbidity and mortality. Aminophylline may help with respiratory drive and diaphragmatic strength, but these effects are unpredictable for a given patient, and it is generally employed in the recovery phase. The other interventions might be harmful.

Board Testing Point: Synthesize treatment for a patient with COPD in early respiratory failure.

---

94. Answer: B

Answer: Administration of isoniazid.
Because this man is a health care worker, 10 mm of induration on his PPD is significant. Since he is asymptomatic and has an unremarkable CXR, his status is categorized as "latent tuberculosis." This means he is infected, but his infection is very limited and isolated by his immune system. He is also classified as a recent converter, and his risk of developing active TB over the next two years exceeds his risk of developing INH-induced hepatitis. He should be given INH treatment. You should understand that the previous verbiage of "isoniazid prophylaxis" and "TB exposure" has now been replaced with "isoniazid treatment" and "latent

tuberculosis." We now refer to patients with positive PPD tests who have never before been treated as having "latent tuberculosis."

Board Testing Point: Recommend treatment for a health care worker with latent tuberculosis.

95. Answer: C

Answer: Bronchogenic carcinoma.
Digital clubbing is not typical of chronic emphysema. While it can occur with tuberculosis, this is unusual as a presenting symptom. The lack of abnormalities of the wrist suggests a diagnosis other than arthritis. The pain with gentle pressure suggests periosteal inflammation that is part of hypertrophic pulmonary osteoarthropathy (HPOA), which often accompanies the digital clubbing due to bronchogenic carcinoma.

Board Testing Point: Consider a diagnosis of bronchogenic carcinoma based on history and physical exam.

96. Answer: D

Answer: Schedule for thoracotomy.
The workup of a solitary pulmonary nodule in a smoker presumes that the lesion is cancer until proven otherwise, despite any attractive epidemiologic exposures to infections. He needs to have a tissue diagnosis. Since the lesion is smaller than 2 cm and is peripheral, bronchoscopy would have a limited role. Thoracotomy will be the best intervention. The presence of a pattern of calcification or a prior chest radiograph that shows no change over a 24-month period would allow for observation as a management strategy. Isolated pulmonary nodule workup does not include fungal serology or mycobacteria sputum culture.

Board Testing Point: Determine the appropriate management of a solitary pulmonary nodule in a smoker.

CARDIOLOGY

97. Answer: C

Answer: 20% less likely (90% pre-test, 70% post-test probability of CAD).
This patient has a high pre-test probability of coronary artery disease (90%) given his risk factors, age, sex, and typical nature of his chest pain. In this setting, the pre-test probability of CAD is a major determinant in the value of a stress test; i.e., in patients with high likelihood of CAD, a negative stress test is likely to be a false negative by Bayesian analysis (see diagram below). Similarly, in patients with a low pre-test probability of CAD, a positive stress test is also unlikely to yield helpful information (more likely to be a false positive). In the diagram below, a treadmill test would be most helpful in a patient with an intermediate pre-test probability of CAD:

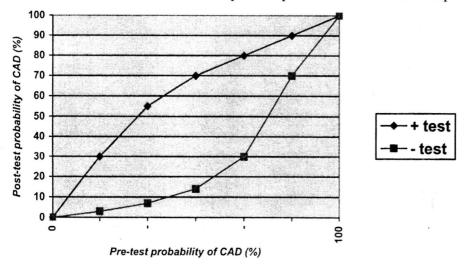

Board Testing Point: Prognosticate the likelihood of true cardiac disease utilizing pre-test probability.

98. Answer: E

Answer: Order an immediate surgical consultation for repair of a ruptured papillary muscle.
Mechanical complications of acute MI include ventricular free wall rupture (< 1%), intraventricular septal rupture (2%), and acute mitral regurgitation. This patient's exam is consistent with mitral regurgitation. Causes of acute mitral regurgitation include LV dilatation, papillary muscle ischemia and papillary muscle chordae rupture. Timing of papillary muscle/chordae rupture is usually 2-7 days post-MI, and presents with hypotension, pulmonary edema, late holo- or mid-systolic murmur (a new murmur in the setting of acute MI). Emergent surgical intervention is necessary because perioperative mortality is 27%. Repeating thrombolytic therapy in this patient is not warranted unless a diagnosis is confirmed. This patient's exam is not consistent with pericardial tamponade or a VSD. RV infarction may present with hypotension but would not lead to pulmonary edema or the murmur described.

Board Testing Point: Diagnose papillary muscle rupture based on physical exam findings and prescribe the appropriate emergent treatment.

99. Answer: E

Answer: Procainamide intravenously.
In patients with underlying structural heart disease/MI, wide complex tachycardia (WCT) is almost always (> 98%) ventricular tachycardia. However, especially in younger patients and/or patients without known heart disease (such as the patient in our question), SVT with aberrancy and WPW/preexcitation must be considered. In patients with VT, though, drugs that treat SVT may cause hemodynamic instability and ventricular fibrillation. Additionally, in patients with preexcitation and atrial fibrillation presenting as wide complex tachycardia, AV nodal blocking agents may cause ventricular fibrillation (by removing the AV nodal protective effect of inhibiting AV conduction, all atrial impulses may travel down the "slick" aberrant pathway and lead to rapid ventricular tachycardia fibrillation). In unstable WCT patients, cardioversion is the treatment of choice. This patient, while anxious, is not unstable. With WCT patients in whom the diagnosis is uncertain, IV procainamide is the initial treatment of choice. Other options include amiodarone, lidocaine, or semi-urgent cardioversion. The correct answer here is procainamide because we cannot say with certainty that this is SVT; it may, in fact, be V. tach from undiagnosed CAD.

Board Testing Point: Identify a wide-complex tachycardia and manage the patient integrating the pertinent history, physical findings and differential diagnosis.

100. Answer: B

Answer: Simvastatin.
Grapefruit juice can increase statin levels markedly, resulting in hepatitis and/or myositis. This is especially true with simvastatin and lovastatin. The other drugs are not affected by grapefruit juice. While not listed as a choice, nifedipine serum levels are also affected by this juice, and patients should be counseled not to ingest grapefruit within an hour of taking nifedipine.

Board Testing Point: Associate grapefruit interactions with statin drugs.

101. Answer: E

Answer: Hemoglobin, ECG.
A baseline hemoglobin measurement is recommended in patients who are undergoing major surgery that is expected to result in significant blood loss (orthopaedic surgery). In healthy patients, there is little rationale to support baseline testing of WBC or platelets. Routine electrolyte determinations are not recommended unless the patient has a history that increases the likelihood of an abnormality (such as renal failure or diuretic use). Routine preoperative tests of hemostasis are not recommended. Their use should be restricted to patients with a known bleeding diathesis or an illness associated with bleeding tendency.

Guidelines for patients in whom routine preoperative ECGs should be obtained:
- Men older than 45 years
- Women older than 55 years
- Known cardiac disease
- Clinical evaluation suggesting the possibility of cardiac disease
- Patients at risk for electrolyte abnormalities, such as diuretic use
- Systemic disease associated with possible unrecognized heart disease, such as diabetes mellitus or hypertension
- Patients undergoing major surgical procedures

This patient has a minor clinical predictor (low-functional capacity) but is scheduled for an intermediate-risk surgery and is over the age of 55, so it is appropriate to order a hemoglobin and ECG prior to surgery. As explained above, another reason to check the hemoglobin is based on the amount of blood loss expected during this specific procedure. In most healthy patients, pre-operative testing should be limited.

With some exceptions (Hb, ECG), preoperative testing should be done only in the setting of known disease or risk factors, and should reflect the underlying disorder.

Board Testing Point: Synthesize an evidence-based, cost-effective pre-operative evaluation.

102. Answer: C

Answer: Complete a risk assessment with dipyridamole thallium test.
This patient is undergoing a high-risk procedure, and both AHA and ACP protocols define him as a moderate-risk patient. Both protocols recommend stress testing prior to surgical planning. A functional test would be more useful than going straight to catheterization. He has atrial fibrillation with a controlled ventricular rate. This patient with atherosclerotic disease undoubtedly has CAD, given his past MI. What is important: Is the myocardium at risk? Cardiac catheterization and TTE would not assess <u>functional</u> status.

Board Testing Point: Do risk assessment of a patient with aortic aneurysm prior to surgery.

103. Answer: E

Answer: Evaluation of the renal arteries with angiography.
This patient most likely has fibromuscular dysplasia (FMD), a non-atherosclerotic cause of renovascular hypertension. FMD is the most common, correctible cause of secondary hypertension and is diagnosed by visualizing a "string of beads" in the distal two-thirds of a renal artery using angiography. Patients who present with hypertension at an early age (< age 30), have the onset of hypertension after the age of 50, have hypertensive urgency/emergency, or have refractory hypertension should be considered good candidates to screen for secondary causes. In patients with renovascular hypertension and typical atherosclerosis risks (hyperlipidemia, family history, smoking, diabetes), atherosclerosis of the renal artery is the most common cause of renovascular hypertension; however, in patients without those risk factors, especially in younger women, FMD must be considered. In addition, the finding of a unilateral abdominal (i.e., renal) bruit also suggests renovascular disease as the cause. This patient has no reason to have renal failure, no risks for diffuse atherosclerosis, and no signs or symptoms of pheochromocytoma, a very rare cause of secondary hypertension. Hyperaldosteronism is a common, reversible cause of secondary hypertension, but in this clinical setting would not be as likely as FMD.

Board Testing Point: Identify the most common cause of secondary hypertension and synthesize the appropriate evaluation.

104. Answer: E

Answer: Echocardiogram.
The history and physical examination suggest the possibility of primary pulmonary hypertension. Pulmonary artery pressures can be estimated by echocardiography. If elevated, then right heart catheterization with monitoring of the response to treatment is warranted. Echo is also necessary to exclude less obvious cardiac causes of secondary pulmonary hypertension. The invasive choices listed (cath, biopsy) are not appropriate. The stress test and the methacholine challenge are not useful in diagnosing pulmonary hypertension.

Board Testing Point: Identify the role of echocardiogram in evaluating possible pulmonary hypertension.

105. Answer: D

Answer: Okay for immediate surgery.
This patient is undergoing nonvascular surgery and is low-to-moderate risk. Neither the AHA nor ACP guidelines would recommend cardiac workup prior to this surgery (thus, no need for Persantine thallium stress test or echocardiogram). His surgery should not be postponed for a transfusion. However, he may well need the transfusion post-operatively.

Board Testing Point: Design a strategy for pre-operative medical clearance for a low-risk surgical procedure.

106. Answer: E

Answer: Propranolol.
Based on his clinical findings of crescendo type angina and the quickly reversible ECG findings of ST-segment elevation, he likely has variant angina (formerly known as Prinzmetal's). The use of the non-selective beta-blocker propranolol has been shown to actually prolong the duration of vasospasm in patients with variant angina. Nifedipine, isosorbide dinitrate, and diltiazem would all be therapeutic and help prevent the spasms. Lovastatin would not help prevent the spasms but would not be contraindicated. Aspirin should be used with caution and is likely best avoided because aspirin inhibits prostacyclin production.

Board Testing Point: Recognize variant angina and prescribe management.

107. Answer: B

Answer: Low voltage of the QRS complexes.
The patient has a pericardial effusion as evidenced by muffled heart tones, distended neck veins and increased pulsus paradoxus, the difference between systolic pressure on inspiration and expiration. A difference of 20 mm Hg or more suggests that the amount of pericardial fluid is sufficient enough to cause cardiac tamponade. Low voltage of the QRS complexes is often associated with tachycardia, ST segment elevation, and T wave changes. None of the other choices is consistent with pericardial effusion.

Board Testing Point: Diagnose cardiac tamponade by physical examination and predict the electrocardiogram findings.

108. Answer: D

Answer: Prolonged PR interval on ECG.
She has rheumatic fever presenting with polyarthritis and erythema marginatum. The diagnosis is suggested by evident improvement of pain with salicylates treatment and rash that is accentuated by fever. Prolonged PR interval is a minor manifestation of rheumatic fever, according to the Jones Criteria. Major manifestations include carditis, polyarthritis, chorea, erythema marginatum (the rash in the picture), and subcutaneous nodules. Minor manifestations include fever, arthralgia, elevated ESR and/or CRP, and prolonged PR interval. The patient must also have supporting evidence of antecedent Group A Streptococcal infection by positive throat culture, rapid antigen detection test, or elevated or increasing streptococcal antibody titer. Increased incidence has occurred in the former Soviet Union. She does not have Lyme disease, Lupus, or bacteremia with *Salmonella*. Joint infection with *Staphylococcus aureus* is very unlikely with her constellation of findings.

Board Testing Point: Identify first-degree heart block as part of the Jones criteria for rheumatic fever.

109. Answer: C

Answer: Slowed carotid upstroke.
This patient has the classic murmur of aortic stenosis. The murmur is best heard at the right upper sternal border and will radiate into the carotid artery. Congenital bicuspid aortic valves usually become calcified and stenotic between the ages of 50 and 70. Usually the normal tricuspid valve will become stenotic at > 80 years of age. A bicuspid aortic valve is the most common inherited valvular disorder and the commonest cause of aortic stenosis. Patients with aortic stenosis will have a "slowed carotid upstroke." "Water-hammer pulse" is seen with chronic aortic regurgitation. Thready pulse is seen with acute aortic regurgitation. Giant right-sided *a* waves are seen with tricuspid stenosis. Bifid pulse is often seen in hypertrophic cardiomyopathy.

Board Testing Point: Identify aortic stenosis by performing a physical exam.

110. Answer: C

Answer: Systemic embolization.
She likely has hyperthyroidism with atrial fibrillation. The longer she has this arrhythmia, the cumulative risk of systemic embolization increases. Atrial fibrillation does not itself provide cumulative risk for any of the other conditions.

Board Testing Point: Recognize the association of hyperthyroidism and atrial fibrillation and the increased risk of systemic thromboembolism.

111. Answer: D

Answer: Electrical cardioversion.
He has ventricular tachycardia and is hemodynamically unstable. He needs immediate cardioversion. Do not attempt medications in a hemodynamically unstable patient with ventricular tachycardia. Overdrive pacing is never an option for this condition. On the general internal medicine examination, assume all wide-complex tachycardia is ventricular tachycardia until proven otherwise!

Board Testing Point: Recognize decompensated ventricular tachycardia and recommend cardioversion.

112. Answer: D

Answer: Amiodarone.
He has hypertrophic cardiomyopathy (HCM). The initial problem in this disorder is diastolic dysfunction. Also, patients with HCM have a tendency for ventricular tachycardias. Young patients with the familial form of the disease are at highest risk for sudden death. Remember that HCM and mitral valve prolapse are the only conditions that have a murmur that INCREASES with standing. To differentiate between the two, do the hand-grip maneuver, because if HCM is present the handgrip maneuver decreases the murmur, while in MVP the maneuver increases the murmur. Anything that decreases left ventricular volume is dangerous in HCM; thus, diuretics, nitrates, and volume depletion are NOT a good idea. Anticoagulants have no place in therapy. Amiodarone is useful to prevent ventricular arrhythmias.

Board Testing Point: Recognize the findings of hypertrophic cardiomyopathy and its increased risk of ventricular arrhythmias with need for treatment.

113. Answer: D

Answer: Admit to the ICU and start intravenous furosemide and an ACE inhibitor.
She has acute heart failure of unknown etiology. In the absence of risk factors for atherosclerosis, the likelihood of coronary artery disease is low in this young woman. Most likely she has viral myocarditis. This is typically seen in young, otherwise healthy individuals and the prognosis is good. With optimal heart failure management, the risk of death or need for acute transplant is low. Therefore, endomyocardial biopsy is reserved for individuals who fail to respond to conventional therapy, develop high-grade heart block, or severe ventricular arrhythmias. There is no reason to start azathioprine or cyclosporine. Hemochromatosis is unlikely given her negative review of systems and ferritin level that is only borderline high; the ferritin may also be borderline because it is an acute phase reactant. It is best to treat her heart failure with standard therapy.

Board Testing Point: Recognize the findings of acute heart failure and prescribe effective therapy.

114. Answer: B

Answer: Echocardiogram.
She has signs and symptoms suggestive of cardiac tamponade: jugular venous distension that is sustained (no collapse during diastole), muffled heart sounds, and decreased amplitude of the QRS complexes. Because this is an emergent presentation, echocardiogram should be done immediately.

Her active urine sediment is consistent with a glomerulonephritis, and her symptoms suggest the onset to be rapidly progressive. The ulcerative purpura is suggestive of Wegener's, a pulmonary-renal syndrome that could be responsible for the concomitant abnormal urine sediment. Likewise, a diagnosis of systemic lupus erythematosus could also be entertained. Antibodies including an ANA, anti-DS DNA and c-ANCA should be performed, but diagnosing the tamponade is more urgent. Pulmonary embolism is unlikely, and therefore neither lower-extremity Doppler ultrasound nor ventilation/perfusion lung scan is indicated.

Board Testing Point: Integrate the history, physical examination, laboratory and electrocardiogram findings to diagnose pericardial tamponade and recommend appropriate diagnostics.

115. Answer: D

Answer: Atrial septal defect.
A 61-year-old woman presents with clinical findings of congestive heart failure secondary to a large left-to-right shunt at the atrial level. ASD is the most common congenital cardiac defect in adults, but frequently does not present as CHF until later in life (age 50-60 years). Women predominate 2-3:1 compared to men. It is not uncommon for patients with ASD to report a heart murmur since childhood and to spontaneously develop atrial fibrillation. The cardiac findings of a fixed split S2 and a murmur at the base of the heart are characteristic. The murmur is due to increased pulmonary blood flow, and not the flow across the ASD. The diastolic murmur is usually secondary to increased flow across the tricuspid valve. Because of the increased volume load on the right side of the heart, the enlarged right atrium and right ventricle are not unexpected. The ECG shows sinus rhythm with right axis deviation, right atrial enlargement (note the peaked P wave in V1) and right ventricular hypertrophy. The procedure of choice would be either surgical or cath-closure of the ASD. None of the other choices are expected in a 61-year-old woman with right-sided heart findings.

Board Testing Point: Diagnose an atrial septal defect in an adult based on history, physical exam and electrocardiogram.

116. Answer: E

Answer: Pulmonic valve stenosis (PS).
He has findings of pulmonic valve obstruction with symptoms of dyspnea and fatigue; the murmur findings listed in his physical examination and his ECG are consistent with PS and are not consistent with any of the other choices. Many patients with moderately severe pulmonary valve stenosis will be asymptomatic in childhood. However, by the time they reach their 20s or 30s, most patients will be symptomatic with dyspnea, shortness of breath, and increased fatigue. Pulmonic valve obstruction needs to be relieved or the symptoms will be progressive.

Board Testing Point: Recognize the findings of pulmonic valve stenosis in an adult.

117. Answer: B

Answer: Left bundle branch block (LBBB).
Note the broadening of the QRS complex <u>and</u> that the abnormality begins from the very first millisecond of ventricular depolarization (as opposed to the "terminal conduction delay" of RBBB). Note also the absence of the septal Q wave in Lead V6! The usual ECG findings are as follows in leads I, V6, and V1:

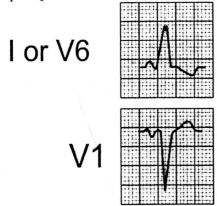

I or V6

V1

Board Testing Point: Recognize the ECG findings of left bundle branch block.

118. Answer: E

Answer: Echocardiogram.
The history and physical examination suggest the possibility of primary pulmonary hypertension. Pulmonary artery pressures can be estimated by echocardiography. If elevated, then right heart catheterization with monitoring of the response to treatment is warranted. Echo is also necessary to exclude less obvious cardiac causes of secondary pulmonary hypertension. The invasive choices listed (cath, biopsy) are not appropriate as initial studies. The stress test and the methacholine challenge are not useful in diagnosing pulmonary hypertension.

Board Testing Point: Recognize the findings of pulmonary hypertension and recommend echocardiogram for evaluation.

119. Answer: D

Answer: Emergent chest x-ray.
Based on the history, elevated blood pressure, and murmur of (new) aortic regurgitation, this patient should be suspected of having an aortic dissection. He is also having a myocardial infarction, which is a known complication of aortic tears that dissect proximally to the coronary arteries. In suspected aortic dissection, rapid imaging is necessary to confirm the diagnosis and to guide therapy, especially in the setting of concomitant MI. Use of thrombolytic therapy is contraindicated in this setting and could be potentially devastating. CXR is usually the initial test, and a wide mediastinum would support the diagnosis. Echocardiography, MRI, CT, or aortography would confirm the diagnosis. Urgent CABG would not be indicated in this setting, nor would pericardiocentesis. High-dose ibuprofen would treat pericarditis, which this patient does not have. Upper endoscopy is not warranted.

Board Testing Point: Recognize and manage aortic dissection.

120. Answer: E

Answer: Perioperative beta-blocker therapy.
Using the Revised Cardiac Risk Index (RCRI), this patient has three significant risk factors for cardiovascular complications during surgery (cerebrovascular disease, insulin-requiring diabetes, creatinine > 2.0 mg/dL); therefore, she has a "compelling indication" for perioperative beta-blocker therapy. Cardiac testing and/or PCI is not necessary in this patient, given the fact that she has not had an MI, and recently underwent cardiac function testing with favorable results. Hemodialysis is not warranted unless she was fluid overloaded or had electrolyte imbalance, and her hemoglobin of 11.2 is appropriate for the operative setting without a need for transfusion. Perioperative ACE inhibitors have not been shown to reduce cardiac complications of surgery; however, beta-blockers have been shown to reduce risk, especially in higher-risk patients ($\geq$ 3 risk factors on the RCRI).

Board Testing Point: Implement appropriate perioperative measures to reduce cardiovascular complications.

121. Answer: B

Answer: A history of untreated strep throat, hemoptysis, and a diastolic rumble at the left 5th interspace at the mid-clavicular line.
This is a pressure tracing of mitral stenosis, showing a diastolic pressure gradient between the left atrium and left ventricle (shaded areas). The most common cause of mitral stenosis is rheumatic fever. Symptoms/signs include atrial fibrillation and elevated pulmonary pressures (symptoms of which may include dyspnea and hemoptysis). Physical findings of mitral stenosis include a diastolic rumble and opening snap. Syncope and a crescendo-decrescendo murmur are characteristic of aortic stenosis. Exertional dyspnea and a holosystolic murmur would suggest mitral regurgitation. CHF, a holosystolic murmur and a positive bubble study indicate a ventricular septal defect. Patients who use IV drugs would be at risk of endocarditis; however, mitral regurgitation rather than stenosis would be the more likely sequela of endocarditis.

Board Testing Point: Identify mitral stenosis by interpreting a left heart pressure tracing.

122. Answer: B

Answer: Glycoprotein IIb/IIIa inhibitor.
In patients with non-ST elevation MI, thrombolytic therapy is not beneficial and should be avoided. Clopidogrel may be used and added to GP IIb/IIIa therapy and heparin in a patient going for PCI, as long as bleeding risk is low. In patients with acute coronary syndromes (ACS) on clopidogrel for whom CABG is expected, clopidogrel should be discontinued for 5 days prior to surgery. Similarly, in ACS patients not on clopidogrel for whom CABG is expected, clopidogrel should be avoided. Immediate-release nifedipine has no role in acute coronary syndromes, and may be harmful because of reflex tachycardia and hypotension. GP IIb/IIIa inhibitors have a Class I indication (level of evidence: A) for patients with NSTEMI who are planned for PCI, and may be used just prior to PCI.

Board Testing Point: Recommend treatment for non-ST elevation myocardial infarction prior to PCI.

123. Answer: A

Answer: One dose of oral amoxicillin prior to the procedure.
Patients who are high-risk should receive endocarditis prophylaxis, and those at moderate risk are usually offered the same. Mitral valve prolapse with an audible murmur of mitral regurgitation, documented mitral regurgitation, or valve leaflet thickening are considered moderate risk for infective endocarditis. Patients at risk and undergoing genitourinary procedures should receive endocarditis prophylaxis. Patients with high-risk conditions should receive intravenous ampicillin plus gentamicin; however, patients with moderate-risk conditions (e.g., MVP plus audible MR murmur) may receive oral amoxicillin (or IV ampicillin) 30 minutes prior to the procedure; gentamicin is not necessary for these patients. The ceftriaxone spectrum is too broad and unnecessary for a simple procedure, and this drug is not recommend in prophylaxis regimens.

Board Testing Point: Recommend antibiotic prophylaxis for infective endocarditis in a patient with mitral valve prolapse and mitral regurgitation undergoing a GU procedure.

124. Answer: B

Answer: Aggressively treat the hypothermia and continue with resuscitation efforts until core temperature is > 33°C (91.4°F).

Terminating resuscitation efforts in a patient who has experienced hypothermia is a difficult clinical decision. The ability of physiological functions to resume at low core body temperatures is very restricted. Treatment of the hypothermia can raise the core temperature, along with the cellular responsiveness to interventions, and increases the potential for success. Unless the core temperature is returned to at least 33° C, cardiac resuscitation should be abandoned only after careful consideration. Brain death evaluation is most appropriate after cardiac and pulmonary status have been stabilized and not in the midst of CPR. Organ harvest in an unidentified patient is inappropriate and should not be implemented until every reasonable effort toward resuscitation has been exhausted.

Board Testing Point: Manage cardiorespiratory arrest secondary to drowning with hypothermia.

125. Answer: B

Answer: A patient with chronic COPD, basilar crepitus and pedal edema presenting with increased shortness of breath.

BNP measurement can help elucidate the presence of congestive heart failure as a component of a patient's clinical status. In a patient with a classic presentation of CHF (elevated JVP, pulmonary congestion, peripheral edema, and an S_3), the BNP is expected to be elevated, and its presence adds nothing to the diagnosis or treatment. The use of the word "brain" in BNP is a historical misnomer, and measurement in the evaluation of a neurologic presentation without evidence of CHF is unnecessary. Likewise, a patient with evidence of renal artery stenosis unassociated with CHF is not an indication to measure BNP. Its greatest clinical utility is in cases where both cardiac and non-cardiac causes can mimic the findings of CHF. Acute shortness of breath may occur with COPD, with CHF, or with both. A low level of BNP is consistent with a pulmonary etiology for the symptoms. An elevated level suggests a cardiac contribution to the presentation.

Board Testing Point: Properly recommend use of brain natriuretic peptide to identify etiologies of shortness of breath.

126. Answer: D

Answer: Aortic dissection.

Marfan syndrome is characterized by: 1) musculoskeletal findings including a tall, thin habitus, spider-like fingers and long extremities, and often with chest and spinal abnormalities; 2) lens displacement (ectopia lentis) with resulting vision disturbances; and 3) aneurysmal disease, most commonly in the aortic root. With this person's physical findings and history of pain consistent with a dissecting aneurysm, prompt evaluation of the thoracic aorta is indicated. Mitral valve prolapse is common in Marfan syndrome but would not account for the acute symptoms, unless it was associated with a dysfunction of the chordae tendineae or papillary muscles. In these circumstances, pulmonary complaints and findings would be much more prominent.

Patients with Marfan syndrome are not exempt from acute pericarditis, myocardial infarction (MI), or pulmonary embolism (PE), but are not at increased risk either. A normal respiratory rate and lack of evidence of thrombotic disease make the diagnosis of PE less likely. The patient lacks a rub on auscultation, the pain is not positional, presented acutely, and has improved without intervention, which makes pericarditis also less likely. The ECG findings are not suggestive of cardiac ischemia. Though it is less likely in this scenario, myocardial ischemia is a common and serious process, and evaluation and intervention for ischemia should proceed concurrently with the evaluation for aortic dissection.

Board Testing Point: Diagnose aortic dissection using history and physical examination; associate Marfan syndrome with aortic dissection.

127. Answer: B

Answer: Patent ductus arteriosus (PDA).
Eisenmenger syndrome is the development of pulmonary hypertension secondary to increased pulmonic blood flow and arises from a left-to-right intracardiac shunt. Over time, the increased flow through the pulmonary vascular beds increases resistance to the point where flow reverses to a right-to-left shunt. This shunt causes significant diversion of unoxygenated blood to the systemic circulation. This can occur with shunts through an atrial septal defect (ASD), a VSD, or a PDA. A VSD can lead to Eisenmenger syndrome, but the cyanosis is more generalized. Critical PS can lead to difficulty with pulmonic blood flow and can demonstrate signs of right heart failure. Similarly, a critical aortic stenosis would exhibit signs of left heart failure. However, neither isolated PS nor isolated AS is associated with cyanosis. A PDA accounts for the findings noted, including the pattern of cyanosis. The differential cyanosis with duskiness to the toes but not to the hands occurs due to the distal insertion of a patent ductus into the aorta. The classic machinery murmur of an untreated PDA is typically altered when the flow of blood is reversed, and there may actually be no murmur at all.

Board Testing Point: Recognize the findings of undiagnosed PDA in a young adult.

128. Answer: D

Answer: Mitral valve prolapse (MVP) with thickened leaflets.
A patient with regurgitant MVP or with thickened leaflets is at an increased risk of endocarditis following dental procedures. The risk from previous CABG and implanted pacemakers and defibrillators is no greater than the risk for the general public. Secundum ASD also lacks an increased risk, whereas an ostium primum ASD is at an increased risk. As long as there are no residua following surgery, and the patient is older than 6 months of age, surgical repair of an ASD, VSD, or PDA does not involve a heightened risk for endocarditis.

Prosthetic valves, a history of previous endocarditis, surgical shunts between the systemic and pulmonary systems, and complex cyanotic congenital heart disease are all high-risk conditions for the development of endocarditis.

Board Testing Point: Recommend appropriate endocarditis prophylaxis.

129. Answer: C

Answer: Her current condition is benign.
Prolapse of the mitral valve is a relatively common finding that is associated with several conditions and can vary significantly in severity. Patients with thickened mitral valves and/or mitral regurgitation are at increased risk of vegetation formation, which in turn raises the risk of embolic phenomenon and the development of endocarditis. Significant mitral regurgitation can result in left ventricular enlargement, but hypertrophy of the left ventricle and sudden death are much more commonly associated with aortic stenosis. MVP with normal leaflets and no regurgitation is most commonly associated with a benign course and may respond symptomatically to beta-blocker therapy. It is not an indication for prophylactic antibiotics.

Board Testing Point: Provide appropriate prognostic counseling to a patient with mitral valve prolapse.

130. Answer: B

Answer: Hypomagnesemia.
Torsade de pointes is a ventricular dysrhythmia with polymorphic QRS complexes. It can arise in many conditions including electrolyte abnormalities, drug interactions, brain injuries, and heart blocks. The most common electrolyte abnormalities associated with torsade de pointes are hypokalemia and hypomagnesemia. Correction of these abnormalities, external pacing control, and beta-blockers are mainstays of therapy. Hyperkalemia, hypocalcemia, and hypernatremia can all affect heart function, but torsade do pointes is not a common feature of these disturbances.

Board Testing Point: Recognize torsades de pointes and the conditions responsible for it.

131. Answer: B

Answer: No swelling or signs of inflammation on right leg exam.
D-dimer is a fibrin degradation product that is produced during a thrombotic process. It is very sensitive to thrombosis, but there are several conditions other than deep vein thrombosis that can result in positive findings on laboratory testing. Pregnancy, malignancy, liver disease, and advanced age can all result in increased D-dimer levels. Technically, these results are not false positives, because the levels are truly elevated but may not arise from an acute thrombosis. In patients with strong evidence of thrombotic disease, a negative D-dimer is too nonspecific to impact treatment decisions. The test is most useful in patients for whom the clinical suspicion of deep venous thrombosis is low. Pain from non-thrombotic conditions may resemble a DVT and a normal D-dimer test would rule against the presence of an acute DVT. Caution must be used, however, because the timing of the D-dimer testing can produce a false-negative test if it is performed either too early or too late in the process.

Board Testing Point: Identify the utility of the D-dimer test in diagnosing acute thromboses.

132. Answer: A

Answer: Amyloidosis.
Restrictive myocarditis arises in several pathological conditions when the heart is infiltrated with abnormal depositions. These include amyloidosis, Fabry disease, hemochromatosis, and sarcoidosis.

Patients with sarcoidosis are uncommonly affected with cardiac manifestations (~5%), whereas lung involvement occurs in nearly 95% of sarcoid patients. A near-normal CXR makes sarcoidosis much less likely.

Abnormal iron deposits are the hallmark of hemochromatosis. These deposits cause dysfunction of the involved organs, and the liver is primarily affected and hepatomegaly is very common. Also, iron pigments in the skin result in a bronzed appearance in the majority (~ 90%) of patients. Cardiac involvement is found in approximately 15% of hemochromatosis patients.

Fabry disease is caused by the absence of an enzyme required for proper metabolism of lipids (*ceramide trihexosidase*). Lipids then accumulate in eyes, kidneys, autonomics and cardiovascular system causing symptoms in adolescence and resulting in death by the fifth decade. Other characteristics include distal paresthesias, lymphedema of the legs, episodic diarrhea, eye opacities, and angiokeratosis. Renal failure often predominates. This patient lacks the neurologic, eye, and bowel problems, which make Fabry disease less likely.

Amyloidosis is one of the more common causes of restrictive myocarditis. It often presents with unexplained proteinuria, CHF, and intermittent abdominal cramping and diarrhea. The findings on echocardiogram are typical of amyloidosis and are referred to as a speckled or diffuse granular pattern. The diagnosis of amyloidosis can be confirmed with biopsy of the oral mucosa or the abdominal subdermal tissue.

Board Testing Point: Integrate findings from the clinical exam to diagnose amyloidosis as an etiology of restrictive myocarditis.

133. Answer: B

Answer: Intravenous ceftriaxone
Lyme disease is caused by the spirochete *Borrelia burgdorferi* and has a wide spectrum of pathology. The rash, erythema migrans, is pathognomonic for the disease, but is not present in every patient or goes either unrecognized or mislabeled, as in this patient. Other possible symptoms include generalized malaise and joint or muscle complaints. More serious disease may include cardiac and neurologic involvement. Oral treatments are adequate for most presentations of Lyme disease, but third-degree heart block and significant neurological disease are best treated by IV antibiotics including ceftriaxone. Oral cephalexin at that stage would not be adequate. Temporary pacing may be necessary, but most heart block from Lyme disease resolves over a relatively short period of time. Kawasaki disease, but not Lyme disease, is associated with coronary artery aneurysms.

Board Testing Point: Be aware that Lyme disease can cause cardiac conduction delays and requires therapy with an IV 3rd generation cephalosporin.

134. Answer: A

Answer: Labetalol.
Acute cocaine intoxication leads to a hyperadrenergic state with potentially life-threatening cardiovascular effects. Propranolol blocks the beta components of these effects but leaves an unopposed alpha effect, which can have significant adverse consequences. Labetalol is able to block both the alpha and beta effects and is the best choice of the medications listed. Nifedipine and enalapril may both affect the blood pressure but do not address the fundamental adrenergic stimulus for the blood pressure elevation and are not the preferred agents. Nifedipine is also associated with increased risk of seizures and mortality in this circumstance.

Board Testing Point: Recommend treatment for cocaine-induced hypertension.

135. Answer: C

Answer: Golf.
He has long QT syndrome. The QT interval is normally (corrected for heart rate) between 340-430 ms. To give you an idea if QT interval lengthening is occurring, look at the R-R interval: the QT interval should be less than 50% of the R-R interval. You can see that the QT interval in this tracing is much longer than ½ of the RR interval. Long QT interval syndrome can be a life-threatening condition that may produce serious dysrhythmias. Strenuous exercise can trigger episodes, which exclude most of the aerobic athletic sports including soccer, badminton, and basketball. In addition, swimming by itself is also noted to occasionally trigger dysrhythmic degeneration. Diving puts a participant at risk of falling from heights if an event occurs on the board and the risk of drowning if an event occurs in the pool. Cricket, golf, and bowling have limited physical exertion and occur in venues where loss of consciousness doesn't include an independent risk of trauma.

Board Testing Point: Recognize the risks of arrhythmias occurring during exercise with long QT syndrome.

136. Answer: A

Answer: Cardiac perfusion studies.
This patient's complaints are highly suggestive of cardiac ischemia and are consistent with cardiac syndrome X. In this condition, the patient experiences ischemia related to microvascular dysfunction in the cardiac tissue with poor blood flow reserve. They often have unremarkable coronary vessel lesions. Accurate diagnosis is vital. Perfusion studies will demonstrate defects and often correlate with ST depressions.

Exercise reproduced her symptoms without significant ectopy. EPS is not indicated without evidence of serious dysrhythmias. Likewise, symptoms exclusively during exercise make a GI source less likely, and a cardiac diagnosis should be fully evaluated before non-lethal, non-cardiac diseases are pursued. Symptoms occurring only with exercise, with a lack of hypertensive findings and adrenergic symptoms make a pheochromocytoma less likely. There is no indication for psychiatric referral in this patient.

Board Testing Point: Recognize the findings in cardiac syndrome X.

137. Answer: B

Answer: Radiofrequency ablation of the accessory pathway.
Preexcitation syndrome occurs when an alternate pathway exists for the conduction of electrical impulses from the atria to the ventricles. Classically (95%), this presents with a short PR interval, a widened QRS complex, and a slurred upswing in the initial R wave (delta wave). Much more uncommonly, the conduction follows the accessory pathway and reenters through the normal pathway. This condition predisposes to episodes of tachycardia and can degenerate to ventricular tachycardia. Digitalis is contraindicated in these circumstances due to its tendency to worsen the condition. Propranolol can be effective when the conduction is primarily through the normal pathway but is of limited value when the primary conduction is through the accessory pathway. The patient's poor adherence also reduces the likelihood that oral medications would provide long-term control. A pacemaker can control the ventricular tachydysrhythmias but predisposes to atrial fibrillation. Both surgical and radiofrequency ablation can effectively provide long-term treatment of this condition, but radiofrequency ablation is safer and more cost-effective. Surgical ablation is reserved for cases that cannot be treated with other modalities.

Board Testing Point: Determine the appropriate therapy for an accessory pathway.

138. Answer: C

Answer: Angina and isosorbide dinitrate.
Significant hypotension is a serious complication that is recognized when sildenafil is used in combination with nitrate medications. Due to the risk, this combination is to be actively avoided. Although the other conditions all have significant morbidity associated with them, the adverse event risk when combined with sildenafil is much less than that noted with nitrates.

Board Testing Point: Identify contraindications for use of sildenafil in a patient with cardiac disease.

139. Answer: D

Answer: B vitamin supplements.
Homocystinemia can arise in several situations, including nutritional deficiencies, medication side effects, and as a genetically based condition. High levels of serum homocysteine have been linked to early-onset cardiovascular disease. Levels of homocysteine can be significantly improved with the use of B vitamin supplements, particularly B-12, B-6, and folate. Propranolol, statins, aspirin, and nitrates all have their role in treating patients following a myocardial infarct, but none of them specifically reduce the levels of circulating homocysteine.

Board Testing Point: Recognize the significance of an elevated homocysteine level and how to lower it with therapy.

140. Answer: C

Answer: Smoking cessation.
Claudication stems from peripheral vascular compromise. The use of dipyridamole has come under scrutiny, and its benefit at this time is very suspect. Support stockings have no role in the treatment of claudication and may actually worsen symptoms. Referral for invasive procedures is more appropriate when surgical intervention is indicated. The indications for surgical intervention in lower extremity peripheral vascular disease include non-healing ulcers, rest pain, and claudications that interfere with the requirements of daily living. At this point, the patient experiences symptoms but is still able to complete his duties. Rest is actually counterproductive, and patients are to be encouraged to exercise to the point of toleration to encourage the development of collateral circulation. The best intervention for this stage of disease is aggressive efforts toward smoking cessation.

Board Testing Point: Recommend tobacco cessation for treatment of claudication.

141. Answer: B

Answer: Severe claudication.
Exercise stress testing is useful for identifying patients with impaired cardiac perfusion. Patients with ischemia exhibit typical ECG findings that aid in the diagnosis of coronary artery disease. Several conditions interfere with the ability of the test to demonstrate the usual changes in the ECG tracing. Among these are bundle branch blocks, pacemaker-driven rhythms, and baseline ST interval changes. The effects of digoxin also interfere with the ECG identification of ischemia. These conditions often require the addition of perfusion or echocardiogram studies.

Severe claudication often restricts individuals from achieving sufficient coronary activity to induce ischemia but does not interfere with the ECG findings. Pharmacologic stress testing can be performed in patients who cannot exercise adequately. A diabetic with no other complicating conditions should be able to perform a conventional exercise ECG study and should not require the use of a pharmacologic agent to stress the heart.

Board Testing Point: Identify situations when pharmacologic stress testing is warranted.

142. Answer: C

Answer: Give fibrinolytic therapy if not contraindicated and if primary percutaneous intervention is not immediately available.
He has likely had an acute myocardial infarction with new LBBB. His ECG shows LBBB with a QRS duration > 120 msec. There is delayed intrinsicoid deflection time in I and V6. There is a monophasic R wave in I.

You should give him ASA, beta-blockers, nitrates prn, and GP IIB/IIIa inhibitor, then monitor his rhythm. If available, he should go for primary percutaneous intervention; if not available, fibrinolytic therapy is indicated. The percutaneous intervention is best if performed within 12 hours of onset of symptoms and within 90 minutes of the arrival of the patient to the ER.

Board Testing Point: Manage an acute MI with new LBBB.

---

143. Answer: C

Answer: Once symptoms develop with aortic stenosis, prognosis is poor.
A bicuspid aortic valve is very common, occurring in 1/50. AS develops two decades earlier in patients with bicuspid valves than those with tricuspid valves. Sudden death occurs in 10% of patients, almost all of whom are symptomatic. A systolic thrill, if it occurs, is located in the suprasternal notch or carotids.

Board Testing Point: Characterize the properties of aortic stenosis.

---

144. Answer: C

Answer: QTc interval.
The phenomenon of torsade de pointes is in reality a special form of polymorphic ventricular tachycardia, wherein the QRS axis appears as if it is twisting around a central perpendicular axis. This is imaginative and not necessarily what is happening in the true spacial sense, but the colorful description is embraced by all admiringly with respect to those who first described it. Torsade de pointes occurs in the setting of prolonged QT interval.

Board Testing Point: Recognize that torsade de pointes is associated with prolonged QT interval.

---

145. Answer: D

Answer: Systemic embolization.
Hyperthyroidism is a well-known cause of atrial fibrillation. As long as the arrhythmia persists, the risk of systemic emboli accumulates. Atrial fibrillation by itself does not increase the risk of any of the other conditions listed, but may be a consequence of some of these other conditions.

Board Testing Point: Recognize atrial fibrillation in a patient with hyperthyroidism and associate an increased risk of systemic embolization.

---

146. Answer: A

Answer: Prominent α and ν waves with hepatomegaly.
This is a case of systemic lupus erythematosus (SLE) causing pulmonary hypertension and high right-sided pressures. The correct answer requires knowledge of how pulmonary hypertension affects venous waveforms. Venous waveforms reflect phases of the cardiac cycle, as seen from "the opposite direction" (i.e. in the venous system, proximal in the vasculature to where contractions are occurring.) The *a* wave results from atrial contraction, and the *x* descent results from atrial relaxation. A smaller *v* wave occurs in atrial diastole as the atrium fills with blood against a closed tricuspid valve (ventricular systole). This is followed by a *y* descent when the tricuspid valve opens and atrial blood fills the ventricle before ventricular systole. Canon *a* waves are seen during periods of AV dissociation, when the asynchronous right atrium attempts to contract against a closed tricuspid valve, and the atrial blood volume rushes back into the jugular vein. Canon *A* waves appear as random

and irregular and are thus distinguished from normal *a* waves. Equal *a* and *v* waves and a low voltage electrocardiogram would occur in cardiac tamponade. Giant *a* waves and a blunted *y* descent occur in settings where the blood flow isn't permitted in an antegrade fashion, and thus goes backward into the venous system, as in the setting of tricuspid stenosis. The jugular venous wave forms would not be normal in the setting of pulmonary hypertension with elevated right-sided pressures causing peripheral edema.

Board Testing Point: Recognize how pulmonary hypertension affects the jugular venous waveform.

147. Answer: D

Answer: Tamponade.
Note that the diastolic pressure in the RA, diastolic pressure in the PA, and PCWP are all the same. The systemic BP is low. Be on the lookout for tamponade in a patient with cancer who suddenly presents decompensated. None of the other choices will give you these values.

Board Testing Point: Interpret pulmonary artery pressures and recognize the findings of tamponade.

148. Answer: C

Answer: Mitral stenosis.
Her physical findings are classic for mitral stenosis. Remember that the symptoms may not show up for many years and frequently are heralded with atrial fibrillation. On the Board exam, also look out for the pregnant woman with mitral stenosis who presents with pulmonary edema, bloody frothy sputum and onset of atrial fibrillation.

Board Testing Point: Identify mitral stenosis by interpreting physical examination findings.

149. Answer: A

Answer: Acute pericarditis.
Note on the ECG the widespread ST segment elevation and PR segment depression, particularly in lead II. NSAIDs are the treatment of choice. A pericardial friction rub is diagnostic as well.

Board Testing Point: Recognize the findings of acute pericarditis.

150. Answer: B

Answer: Initiate pacing because this is 3rd degree AV block.
With this condition, there is no conduction between the atria and the ventricles. Permanent pacing is indicated in most patients, but temporary pacing can be initiated until the etiology can be sorted out. This is not due to an "allergic" reaction to beta-blockers. You see progressive prolongation of the PR interval until there is a dropped QRS in 2° AV block type 1.

Board Testing Point: Recognize 3rd degree AV block and the necessity for pacing.

151. Answer: D

Answer: Wolff-Parkinson-White syndrome (WPW).
Note the delta waves. The PR interval is short < 120 ms, and the ECG has a prolonged QRS complex. Remember that AV nodal blockers should be avoided because they may accelerate conduction through the accessory pathway. IV procainamide or cardioversion are the treatments of choice. Definitive therapy is catheter ablation.

Board Testing Point: Recognize WPW syndrome based on history and electrocardiogram.

152. Answer: D

Answer: Enalapril.
Remember she is pregnant! Of the drugs listed, only enalapril is contraindicated in pregnancy; enalapril is associated with teratogenicity. The other agents, as well as electrical cardioversion, are deemed "OK" during pregnancy. Other contraindicated agents commonly queried on the Board in pregnant patients are ciprofloxacin, warfarin, nitroprusside, doxycycline, and valproic acid.

Board Testing Point: Identify enalapril as contraindicated in pregnancy.

153. Answer: B

Answer: Tricyclic overdose.
Tricyclic overdose is most consistent with prolonged QT intervals. Of the choices, hyperkalemia would not cause a prolonged QT interval (but hypokalemia does). Hypocalcemia, hypomagnesemia, and a liquid protein diet would as well. Other etiologies include starvation, CNS insult, erythromycin, and ischemia.

Board Testing Point: Recognize conditions that prolong the QT interval.

154. Answer: C

Answer: Risk assess with dipyridamole thallium test.
This patient is undergoing a high-risk procedure, and both AHA and ACP protocols define him as a moderate-risk patient. Both protocols recommend stress testing prior to surgical planning. A functional test would be more useful than going straight to catheterization. A standalone TTE is not going to be useful in risk assessment. This high-risk patient with atherosclerotic disease undoubtedly has CAD, given his past MI. What is important: is the myocardium at risk?

Board Testing Point: Evaluate and recommend appropriate pre-operative assessment.

155. Answer: E

Answer: Neurocardiogenic (vasovagal) syncope.
Neurocardiogenic vasovagal syncope is the most common cause of syncope in young adults. The history of feeling lightheaded, with tunnel vision, while standing is typical. The other entities can also present with syncope, but are far less common. As many as 16% of individuals will faint at least once in their lives. The other choices are rare in young, healthy people, and without physical findings it would not be useful to embark on a major diagnostic workup.

Board Testing Point: Recognize vasovagal syncope as the most common cause of syncope in an otherwise healthy, young person.

156. Answer: A

Answer: < 2 μg/kg/min.
Less than 2 μg/kg/min stimulates beta-adrenergic receptors and increases myocardial contractility. 2-5 μg/kg/min stimulates beta-adrenergic receptors and increases renal blood flow. > 10 μg/kg/min has mainly alpha-agonist effects and causes vasoconstriction. The Boards occasionally will ask a straightforward pharmacology question like this.

Board Testing Point: Characterize the dose-dependent effects of dopamine.

157. Answer: E

Answer: Hypertrophic cardiomyopathy.
This patient has hypertrophic cardiomyopathy (HCM), which is the most common cause of sudden death in exercising young people. Abnormal coronary arteries are the next most common disorder, but they do not demonstrate the same abnormalities on physical exam as HCM. No medications have been shown to prolong survival only heart transplant. Beta-blockers and verapamil will improve symptoms, however. The carotid pulse finding in this disorder is also seen in aortic stenosis, but the history and murmur are characteristic of HCM. Mitral valve prolapse would not produce these findings either.

Board Testing Point: Recognize the findings of hypertrophic cardiomyopathy.

158. Answer: D

Answer: Observation only.
He has Mobitz I or Wenckebach pattern of 2nd degree heart block. In this pattern, there is a cycle of progressive prolongation of the PR interval until the QRS complex is dropped. Mobitz I 2nd degree heart block does not progress to complete heart block as can Mobitz II (unchanging PR intervals in the conducted beats). He is asymptomatic and does not require a temporary pacemaker. If he had a Mobitz type II heart block, a permanent pacemaker would be indicated. An ACE inhibitor is not indicated.

Board Testing Point: Recognize the differences between Mobitz I and II heart block.

159. Answer: A

Answer: Immediate synchronized cardioversion.
This man is in moderate distress with hypotension and has likely ventricular tachycardia on ECG. He requires immediate synchronized cardioversion. Because of the distress and the hypotension, pharmaceutical agents are not first-line therapy. For the ABIM exam, always cardiovert any symptomatic patient with a dysrhythmia.

Board Testing Point: Identify a wide-complex tachycardia and manage the patient integrating the pertinent history, physical findings and differential diagnosis.

160. Answer: E

Answer: Long-acting nitrates and diltiazem.
This is a case of variant angina. In support of this diagnosis: history of rest pain, ST depression that rapidly resolves and is not associated with the release of cardiac enzymes, and normal coronary arteries. No arrhythmia was noted during the event, so lidocaine is not justified. However, syncope associated with variant angina is often due to occasional ventricular arrhythmias, so careful monitoring is warranted. The normal cardiac catheterization excludes unstable angina, so treatment for acute coronary syndromes is unnecessary. Long-acting nitrates and calcium channel blockers are effective in reducing the numbers of events of vasospasm in cases of variant angina.

Board Testing Point: Recognize the syndrome of variant (Prinzmetal) angina and implement appropriate management.

161. Answer: D

Answer: Order an immediate surgical consultation for repair of a ruptured papillary muscle.
A similar question was asked elsewhere, but we've asked it again just to reemphasize that this is an important complication of acute MI to recognize! It will appear on your Board Examination!

Mechanical complications of acute MI include ventricular free wall rupture (< 1%), intraventricular septal rupture (2%), and acute mitral regurgitation. This patient's exam is consistent with mitral regurgitation. Causes of acute mitral regurgitation include LV dilatation, papillary muscle ischemia and papillary muscle chordae rupture. Timing of papillary muscle/chordae rupture is usually 2-7 days post-MI, and presents with hypotension, pulmonary edema, late holo- or mid-systolic murmur (a new murmur in the setting of acute MI). Emergent surgical intervention is necessary because perioperative mortality is 27%. Repeating thrombolytic therapy in this patient is not warranted unless a diagnosis is confirmed. This patient's exam is not consistent with pericardial tamponade or a VSD. RV infarction may present with hypotension but would not lead to pulmonary edema or the murmur described.

Board Testing Point: Diagnose papillary muscle rupture based on physical exam findings and prescribe the appropriate emergent treatment.

162. Answer: D

Answer: Atrial flutter.
Usually atrial flutter occurs at an atrial rate of 220-320 with the ventricular rate being an even number division of the atrial rate. There is usually a "sawtooth" pattern in II, III, aVF, and V1. Vagal maneuvers can slow the ventricular response. Her ventricular response is too regular to be atrial fibrillation. She has no evidence of 2nd degree heart block (prolonged PR interval with dropping of a QRS), and 3rd degree heart block is not consistent with this ECG.

Board Testing Point: Recognize the ECG findings of atrial flutter.

163. Answer: C

Answer: Intravenous fluid resuscitation.
This patient is suffering from acute right heart failure secondary to an acute right ventricular infarction, a condition which complicates approximately 25% of inferior myocardial infarcts. Electrocardiographic evidence of inferior wall infarction includes ST segment elevation in leads II, III and aVF, and ST elevation in lead V1. Right-sided chest leads, when performed, usually demonstrate ST elevation. She has recognizable signs of severe RV failure such as Kussmaul's (an increase in jugular venous pressure with inspiration, owing to a poorly compliant right ventricle and impaired filling), hepatic congestion, and slow-to-resolve hepatojugular reflux. These patients may or may not have hypotension. With a failing right ventricle, left ventricular filling pressures are entirely dependent on preload. Hence, patients with an acute inferior MI are sometimes made worse with medications that reduce preload, such as nitroglycerin. The patient's heart rate is too low to tolerate labetalol. This low rate could be a direct consequence of SA node infarction. Because the left ventricle is not failing, an inotrope is unnecessary, and the diuretic will also reduce preload. Nesiritide is approved only for use in decompensated congestive heart failure. While angiography would be advised in this case, the next most appropriate management is to increase the patient's preload and blood pressure with intravenous fluids. Patients with right ventricular infarction as a complication of an inferior wall STEMI have a much worse prognosis than patients with isolated inferior wall STEMI.

Board testing point: Implementation of the appropriate treatment of severe right ventricular failure during inferior myocardial infarction.

164. Answer: B

Answer: 1st degree AV block.
Note the prolonged PR interval but no lengthening of the PR interval or dropping of a QRS after a P wave.

165. Answer: C

Answer: 2nd degree AV block, Mobitz I.
Note the gradual prolonging of the PR interval with the eventual dropping of a QRS complex. This leads to "grouped beating" of QRS complexes. There is always one more P wave than QRS complexes in each group. The only indication for treatment is symptomatic bradycardia.

166. Answer: D

Answer: 2nd degree AV block, Mobitz II.
Note that the PR interval is not lengthening and that a QRS just "drops out." In this case, "group beating" is seldom present. This type of block is more likely to progress to 3rd-degree block than Mobitz I. Pacing is indicated in symptomatic patients.

167. Answer: D

Answer: Atrial fibrillation.
Note the irregularly irregular QRS pattern as well as the lack of easily identifiable P-waves. The atrial rate is between 400-600. Most cases appear to arise from the distal pulmonary veins as they insert into the left atrium. Vagal maneuvers or adenosine slow the ventricular response.

168. Answer: C

Answer: Atrial flutter.
Note the "saw-toothed" pattern of P-waves. This is classic atrial flutter. The atrial rate is usually between 220-320 and the ventricular rate is usually an even number division of the atrial rate. There is usually a saw-tooth pattern in II, III, aVF, and V1. Every regular SVT with a rate of 150 is atrial flutter with 2:1 block until proven otherwise. Vagal maneuvers will slow ventricular response.

169. Answer: D

Answer: Left bundle branch block.
Criteria for left bundle branch block (LBBB) include the following:
1) QRS = 120-180 ms (3-4.5 small squares)
2) The left ventricle is depolarized later resulting in an RR' (slurred or notched) in V6 and an SS'(QS) in V1
3) The T wave is often opposite the mean QRS vector in anteroseptal and lateral leads

170. Answer: E

Answer: Right bundle branch block.
Criteria for right bundle branch block (RBBB) include:
1) QRS > 120 ms (3 small squares)
2) Depolarization of the right ventricle is delayed resulting in an RSR' ("rabbit ears") or RR' in V1 and often a slurred S wave in V5-6.
3) Flipped T waves in V1, sometimes V2.

171. Answer: D

Answer Inferior MI.
Note the ECG changes in II, III, and aVF.

Septal MI = changes in V1-2
Anterior MI = changes in V3-4
Anteroseptal MI = V1-4
Lateral MI = I, aVL, V6
Anterolateral = I, aVL, V3-6 (extensive will involve V1-V6!)
Inferior = II, III, aVF
Apical = II, III, aVL and any of V1-V4
Posterior = Tall R in V1-2
High lateral = I, aVL

172. Answer: B

Answer: Anterolateral MI.
This patient has ECG changes in I, aVL, and V1-V6 indicating an EXTENSIVE anterolateral MI.

Septal MI = changes in V1-2
Anterior MI = changes in V3-4
Anteroseptal MI = V1-4
Lateral MI = I, aVL, V6
Anterolateral = I, aVL, V3-6 (extensive will involve V1-V6!)
Inferior = II, III, aVF
Apical = II, III, aVL and any of V1-V4
Posterior = Tall R in V1-2
High lateral = I, aVL

173. Answer: D

Answer: Wolff-Parkinson-White (WPW).
In WPW, an accessory pathway allows early depolarization of some part of the ventricle, producing delta waves. WPW invalidates the interpretation of old MIs and LVH. WPW can be associated with narrow or wide complex tachycardias. Here the delta waves are very noticeable in I and aVL. Note the following diagram for a better explanation.

WPW

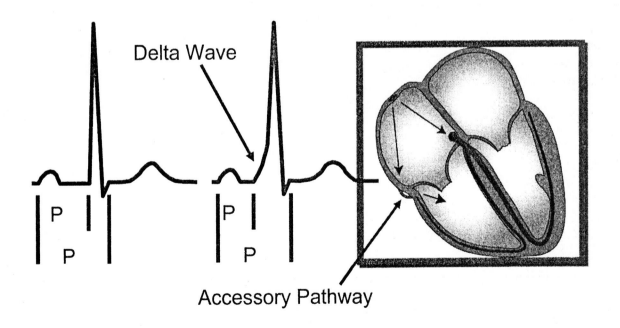

174. Answer: C

Answer: Pericarditis.
Recognize and note the diffuse ST segment elevation! Note also the PROMINENT PR segment depression, most notably in lead II! This is the classic ECG for pericarditis.

175. Answer: D

Answer: Ventricular tachycardia.
For goodness sakes know this one! If the patient is unstable, SHOCK! If the patient is stable, you can use medications like procainamide.

176. Answer: D

Answer: Reassurance.
Isolated PVCs or even trigeminy as in this patient are almost always benign in a healthy young person. They generally require no therapy or evaluation!

INFECTIOUS DISEASES

177. Answer: C

Answer: Trimethoprim-sulfamethoxazole.
Community-acquired methicillin-resistant *S. aureus* (MRSA) is an emerging challenge for infection control. These strains are often associated with skin and soft tissue infections, but may also cause sepsis, pneumonia, and necrotizing pathology. Clindamycin, trimethoprim-sulfamethoxazole, and quinolones are outpatient options for oral treatment. Unfortunately, community-acquired MRSA has a significant tendency to develop inducible resistance to both clindamycin and the quinolones. The erythromycin-clindamycin D-zone test evaluates an MRSA isolate for its capacity to express inducible resistance genes in the presence of clindamycin. A positive D-zone test indicates that even though an isolate appears susceptible to clindamycin *in vitro*, the organisms can express their resistance genes after being in the presence of clindamycin after some time. Thus, clindamycin is inappropriate as a prescription in the setting of a positive D-zone test.

Unfortunately, we have no such test for the quinolone drugs. Should you choose to treat an MRSA skin infection with a quinolone, you must be vigilant in observing the clinical response to ensure treatment failure does not occur. Gatifloxacin is contraindicated in diabetics because of dangerous blood glucose derangements. Vancomycin requires intravenous administration, and is unnecessary for skin and soft tissue infections only (in the absence of osteomyelitis.) MRSA is resistant to dicloxacillin.

Board Testing Point: Design a treatment regimen for a skin and soft tissue infection with community-acquired methicillin-resistant *Staphylococcus aureus* integrating the D-zone test result.

178. Answer: B

Answer: Toxic shock syndrome toxin 1.
Toxic shock syndrome is a toxin-mediated process resulting from infection with either a toxin-producing *Staphylococcus aureus* or *Streptococcus pyogenes*. Although initially associated with tampon usage, current presentations can arise from any infection due to Staph or Strep organisms. Absence of host antibodies to the circulating toxin appears to be a primary risk for developing a toxic shock presentation. Treatment requires prompt intravenous fluid support, identification of the primary infection locus, and aggressive treatment of the underlying infection, including drainage of any localized purulence. Pending cultures, treatment is optimized with a beta-lactamase-resistant, anti-staphylococcal antibiotic in combination with clindamycin. Clindamycin inhibits protein synthesis, which reduces the production of toxins and cytokines contributing to the systemic findings. Bacteria in deep-tissue abscesses are often in a stationary phase of growth, and very few organisms are replicating; hence, beta-lactam drugs that act on the cell wall during logarithmic growth are not the most effective drugs. Adding clindamycin helps to kill these organisms in stationary phase.

Desquamation, which is common in this disease process, is often delayed by 10-14 days from the original presentation.

Both Steven-Johnson syndrome and toxic epidermal necrolysis are often caused by severe drug reactions that affect epidermal integrity resulting in varying degrees of epidermal detachment. Both can affect internal organs as well, resulting in a poor prognosis. This rash was present before the onset of medications and is not consistent with either of these diagnoses.

Staphylococcal scalded skin syndrome (SSSS) is mediated by two types of toxin: exfoliative toxin A and exfoliative toxin B. It is more common in younger children and displays blister formation often with severe exfoliation. The skin is often tender to palpation, and the mucous membranes are usually spared.

Erysipelas is a superficial infection limited to the epidermis typically caused by beta-hemolytic streptococci. The presence of the rash is typically concurrent with systemic symptoms, if these are present. Erysipelas is generally well-demarcated with raised edges, brightly erythematous, and tender to the touch. Rarely are systemic symptoms associated.

Board Testing Point: Differentiate among the various etiologies of shock with desquamation; identify toxic shock syndrome toxin 1 as critical to the disease process of toxic shock syndrome.

179. Answer: D

Answer: Topical permethrin.
Scabies is a parasitic infestation from the mite *Sarcoptes* scabies, which causes an extremely pruritic rash. Burrows (as seen in the hand picture) are commonly noted. Transmission can readily occur from person to person, and outbreaks are possible in long-term care facilities, hospitals, and mental institutions. Patients with decreased mental status, compromised immune function, and glucocorticoid usage are at risk for hyper-infestation, resulting in a variant referred to as Norwegian scabies. This form is extensive and associated with diffuse crusting, as described in this patient's roommate. The responsible mite can be effectively eliminated by the use of permethrin. Itching often continues after the removal of the offending mites due to persistence of fecal pellets, which continues until the skin containing these pellets is replaced during normal dermal turnover. Oral antibiotics may be necessary for secondary bacterial involvement, but that is not described in this scenario. Topical steroids, oral diphenhydramine, and calamine lotion can provide symptomatic relief but have no effect on eradicating the offending mite.

Board Testing Point: Analyze the presentation of scabies in a nursing home setting and prescribe appropriate treatment.

180. Answer: C

Answer: Td in combination with tetanus immune globulin (TIG).
Tetanus (lockjaw) is a neurologic disease mediated by a neurotoxin produced by the anaerobe *Clostridium tetani*. This organism is ubiquitous, but is more common in wounds contaminated with dirt, feces, or saliva. Patients with burns and wounds that compromise dermal defenses (penetrating or desquamating processes) are at an increased risk of tetanus. Patients who have not completed the primary vaccination series or patients with serious wounds and an unknown immunization status should receive both the appropriate tetanus toxoid vaccine **and** TIG. Use of DTaP is restricted to children younger than 7 years of age, while individuals older than 7 years of age should receive Td. There are no contraindications to the coadministration of tetanus vaccine and tetanus immune globulin, except that they must be given in different body sites. With the recent FDA approval of Tdap, which includes an acellular pertussis component, future answers may include this as a choice for adults, but currently it is not indicated.

Board Testing Point: Construct a vaccine regimen to protect against tetanus for a non-immunized patient with multiple contaminated wounds.

181. Answer: A

Answer: Emergent surgical exploration and debridement.
Necrotizing fasciitis is a rapidly progressive infection that tracks through the subcutaneous tissues and fascial planes. Early recognition and prompt intervention is essential to improve outcome and reduce mortality. Mixed aerobe/anaerobic infections, Clostridia, and *S. pyogenes* are frequently implicated in the process. Clostridia infections are noted for the frequent development of gas gangrene in the affected tissues. Gas gangrene, however, is not universally present. CT scans may delineate the extent of involvement but often only show nonspecific swelling. The presence of violaceous blisters suggests a very severe underlying deep tissue infection. Leading-edge aspiration and biopsy are often unrevealing. Surgical intervention permits necessary debridement and allows for microbiologic identification of the responsible etiologies. Antibiotics without debridement are inadequate to contain most cases of necrotizing fasciitis.

Board Testing Point: Recognize necrotizing fasciitis based on clinical history and physical examination, and make an urgent surgical referral.

182. Answer: A

Answer: Oral mebendazole.
This presentation is typical for infection with *Enterobius vermicularis* (pinworms). Pinworms are a parasitic infection, with humans as the only natural host. The females perpetuate the life cycle by laying eggs in the perianal area. Irritation caused by the worms stimulates scratching, which transfers the eggs to the fingers and then to the mouth to continue the GI infestation. The "scotch tape" test involves placing a piece of scotch tape on the anus, then removing it and looking for the eggs stuck on the scotch tape under the microscope. Mebendazole (Vermox®) is an effective treatment for this disease, but may require repeat administrations to fully eradicate the pinworms.

Nystatin is used for topical candidiasis; cephalexin would be used for bacterial cellulitis; permethrin is used for a scabies or lice infestation. Hydrocortisone may alleviate many of the local symptoms but would not affect the fundamental process.

Board Testing Point: Recognize the presentation of pinworms and prescribe appropriate therapy.

183. Answer: E

Answer: Td booster, oral amoxicillin/clavulanate after one dose of parenteral antibiotics, no rabies vaccine, consultation with hand surgeon.
Animal bites are often polymicrobial infections (*Staphylococcus sp.*, *Streptococcus sp.*, Gram negatives, and anaerobes) that may include *Pasteurella multocida* (30-50%). Dog bites are usually not as deep as cat bites. Cat teeth are sharper and more slender and may be more likely to extend down to bone. Amoxicillin/clavulanate is the drug of choice for all bites due to a beta-lactamase produced by the *Pasteurella* organism. In this case, with the severity of the bite wound and possible compartment syndrome, it is prudent to give a parenteral antibiotic (such as ampicillin/sulbactam). Bites on the hand require consultation with a hand surgeon because of the chance of rapid spread of infection through fascial planes. All animal bites are considered high risk for tetanus; therefore, anyone without a booster within 5 years should get a Td booster. Rabies shots (post-exposure vaccination) are necessary only if the animal shows signs of illness or if the animal cannot be quarantined.

Board Testing Point: Identify beta-lactamase producing *Pasteurella* as a potential player in a polymicrobial bite wound of the hand and prescribe appropriate antibiotics; prescribe post-exposure prophylaxis for tetanus and rabies in the setting of a domestic animal bite.

184. Answer: B

Answer: Administration of hepatitis B vaccine.
Trimethoprim-sulfamethoxazole can be an effective replacement for ampicillin/sulbactam therapy on penicillin-allergic patients, but should be coupled with clindamycin to provide adequate coverage for the pathogens found in a human bite (specifically *Eikenella*). Wound closure is not indicated in a wound this old. HBIG is not indicated since hepatitis B exposure in this situation is very unlikely. Hepatitis B vaccine, however, is indicated for certain subgroups of the population, including inmates of both juvenile detention and criminal detention facilities. Tetanus booster within 5 years is adequate even for contaminated wounds.

Board Testing Point: Determine the need for vaccination against hepatitis B in high-risk populations.

185. Answer: A

Answer: No antibiotics, remove Foley and peripheral central venous catheters, discharge to home.
Asymptomatic bacteriuria does not require treatment in patients with an indwelling catheter, even in the presence of WBCs in the urine. Patients in whom asymptomatic bacteriuria should be treated include pregnant women, men about to undergo TURP, and patients about to undergo urologic procedures in which mucosal bleeding is anticipated; it also may be considered in asymptomatic women with catheter-acquired bacteriuria that persists 48 hours after indwelling catheter removal. Patients in whom screening for bacteriuria is **not** recommended include the following: premenopausal, nonpregnant women; diabetic women; older persons living in the community; elderly, institutionalized subjects; persons with spinal cord injury; and catheterized patients while the catheter remains *in situ*.

Board Testing Point: Manage asymptomatic bacteriuria in a hospitalized patient with a Foley catheter.

186. Answer: D

Answer: Counsel the patient to abstain from contact sports.
This patient has mononucleosis, most likely EBV-associated. The presence of palatal petechiae, exudative pharyngitis, and a morbilliform rash that worsens after exposure to amoxicillin is highly suggestive of EBV. In addition, he has an enlarged spleen on physical exam, which makes him susceptible to splenic rupture. All significantly ill patients with EBV should be advised to avoid activities that could lead to splenic rupture. A white blood cell count with differential may show atypical lymphocytes, and a heterophile antibody test confirms the diagnosis. There is no reason for this patient to specifically avoid alcohol, sulfa-based drugs, estuarine water exposure, or sun exposure given this history.

Board Testing Point: Associate EBV-associated mononucleosis with splenomegaly, and counsel that contact sports are contraindicated.

187. Answer: C

Answer: Quinine plus doxycycline.
This patient has falciparum malaria. Malaria should be at the top of the diagnostic list for any traveler returning from Africa with fever. The picture is showing a "banana gametocyte," classic for *P. falciparum*. Other diagnostic possibilities include typhoid fever, dengue fever, tuberculosis, leptospirosis, and helminthic diseases. Chloroquine is not appropriate prophylaxis for travelers to most malaria-endemic areas, since chloroquine resistance is high, including in central Africa (see map below, taken from CDC website).

Some chemoprophylaxis regimens require starting medicine prior to the trip and continuing prophylaxis for up to four weeks after returning (e.g., mefloquine). In Africans with partial immunity, chloroquine is often used for treatment of malaria; however, it should not be used for treatment of falciparum malaria in non-immune travelers. Chloroquine + primaquine is the recommended treatment for *P. vivax* and *P. ovale* (primaquine must be used to eradicate the hypnozoites in the liver, which may cause recurrences months after the initial infection). Although *P. vivax* is the most common form of malaria worldwide, the only species of malaria that causes **multiply-infected** erythrocytes is *P. falciparum*. Thus, in this patient with multiple-infected RBCs, the diagnosis is *P. falciparum*, and first-line treatment is quinine plus doxycycline. Exchange transfusion may be used for children and for severe malaria (very high parasite load, at least > 10%), but in stable patients it is not necessary.

(from CDC website: www2.ncid.cdc.gov/travel/yb/utils/ybGet.asp?section=dis&obj=index.htm#map4-6)

Map 4-6. Malaria-endemic countries in the Western Hemisphere

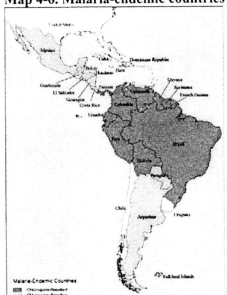

Map 4-7. Malaria-endemic countries in the Eastern Hemisphere

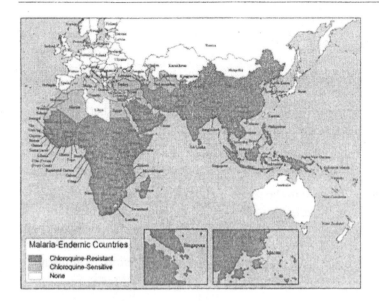

Board Testing Point: Diagnose and compose a treatment regimen for a febrile traveler returning from Africa with probable malaria.

188. Answer: A

Answer: HSV encephalitis.
This patient's symptoms are typical of temporal lobe involvement due to infection with herpes simplex virus (HSV). Symptoms usually are acute in onset, associated with fever, and may include unusual behavior, seizures, dysphasia, amnesia, cranial nerve deficits, and ataxia. Abnormal signal enhancement in the temporal lobe is very suggestive of HSV encephalitis in the proper clinical setting. Temporal lobe epilepsy presents with automatisms, staring episodes, and altered consciousness, but imaging would not show enhancement. Patients with a brain abscess have a more indolent clinical course, complaining of symptoms related to mass effect, and the MRI would show an enhancing focal lesion. Glioblastoma multiforme appears as an irregularly-shaped mass with central necrosis and extensive edema; a completely different appearance from HSV encephalitis. Although patients with HSV encephalitis may exhibit signs of hypomania and unusual behavior, this patient does not fit the criteria for schizoaffective disorder.

Board Testing Point: Diagnose HSV encephalitis using history, physical exam and neuroimaging.

189. Answer: A

Answer: Mefloquine.
DEET is an effective mosquito repellant with limited safety studies in pregnancy. High concentrations of DEET have been linked with rashes, seizures, and encephalopathy in children. Concentrations over 50% have not been shown to provide additional protection. Frequent, direct application of high-concentration DEET to skin is not recommended. Both atovaquone-proguanil and doxycycline are contraindicated in pregnancy. The Committee on Infectious Diseases recommends mefloquine as the drug of choice for pregnant patients in high-risk, chloroquine-resistant malaria situations.

Board Testing Point: Prescribe appropriate malaria prophylaxis to a pregnant patient.

190. Answer: B

Answer: Sickle cell disease.
Meningococci are Gram (-) diplococci with a polysaccharide capsule. *Neisseria meningitides* is responsible for several pathological conditions, including meningococcemia and meningococcal meningitis. Close housing conditions, such as military barracks and college dormitories, as well as travel to endemic areas (the African meningitis belt), are risk factors. As with other encapsulated organisms, asplenia is also a risk factor for meningococcal disease. The vaccine is recommended for asplenic patients, including functional asplenia resulting from sickle cell disease. Individuals with properdin or late complement-component deficiencies also benefit from vaccination with quadrivalent meningococcal polysaccharide vaccine. Chronic asthma, cystic fibrosis, and seizure disorder are not risk factors for acquiring meningococcal disease.

Board Testing Point: Identify the patient groups for which the polysaccharide meningococcal vaccine is recommended.

191. Answer: D

Answer: Counsel that valacyclovir or famciclovir started in the first 48 hours of a zoster flare can reduce the duration of post-herpetic neuralgia.
Varicella zoster is responsible for chicken pox (varicella) in children, herpes zoster in adults, and infrequently, primary varicella infections in adults. Adults who experience a primary infection with varicella tend to have a much more serious course, with increased morbidity and mortality. Primary infection in adults does not present as shingles, but rather presents as a very serious case of chicken pox with possible pneumonia and/or encephalitis. Children can contract varicella from an adult with shingles, but an adult does not contract shingles from a child with chicken pox. Shingles can result only after primary infection of the virus (chickenpox) and after the virus has established itself in the nerve roots. Shingles then results when the virus reactivates at a later date. Dermatomal flares are consistent with reactivation of dormant varicella virus in adults who experienced the initial infection during childhood. Vaccination for susceptible patients older than 12 years of age requires two injections at least one month apart to achieve reasonable levels of immunity. With this vaccine, you are preventing primary infection with chicken pox; and the reason to vaccinate is to prevent the serious morbidity from adult chicken pox. Valacyclovir or famciclovir started early in the course of a zoster flare can reduce the duration of post-herpetic neuralgia. These 2 agents have been shown to be superior to acyclovir.

Board Testing Point: Know the early treatment of varicella zoster and that valacyclovir and famciclovir can reduce the duration of post-herpetic neuralgia.

192. Answer: C

Answer: Start doxycycline and send blood for serology.
This patient has Rocky Mountain Spotted Fever (RMSF). Fevers, arthralgia, and a maculopapular rash that progresses to a petechial rash on the extremities spreading to the trunk are classic signs and symptoms. Patients may also present with diarrhea and abdominal pain. Diagnosis is based on a high index of suspicion and clinical findings, and it is imperative to begin treatment immediately, since this disease does have 3% mortality. Serological testing can be done for confirmation but should not delay treatment. Doxycycline is the treatment of choice for RMSF regardless of age. Definite diagnosis can be obtained via immunofluorescent staining on a biopsy of a petechial lesion, but this too should not delay treatment. Ceftriaxone 2 grams IV q 24 h is the treatment for patients with Lyme disease who are manifesting cardiac and neurologic sequelae and for presumed pneumococcal or meningococcal sepsis. This patient's history of hiking in the mountains, however, makes the possibility of RMSF more likely than either *S. pneumoniae* or *N. meningitidis*.

Board Testing Point: Differentiate among infections that present with fever, rash, and arthralgia; and synthesize a differential diagnosis based on the geographical clues presented.

193. Answer: C

Answer: *Francisella tularensis.*
Combine Missouri, tick exposures, lymphadenopathy, fever, eschar, and a person who frequents the woods, and tularemia is the most likely answer. *Yersinia* would be found in the desert Southwest. There are 14 different species of leptospires that cause disease; infection with any of them would present with fever, headache, and, (frequently tested on the Boards) conjunctival suffusion and an obstructed jaundice picture. *Ehrlichia* is a possibility in this geographic area, but it does not cause a single lymph node enlargement, and you would expect patient to present a CBC showing pancytopenia. *Bordetella pertussis* causes pertussis, a respiratory disease that has nothing to do with this presentation.

Board Testing Point: Diagnose tularemia using the history and physical exam; integrate epidemiology into the differential diagnosis of an infectious disease.

194. Answer: B

Answer: *Staphylococcus aureus.*
She meets criteria for a diagnosis of toxic shock syndrome due to *S. aureus*. Note the question mentions "menses." If you see menses mentioned in a question with possible infection, think of two scenarios: 1) Toxic shock syndrome and 2) Disseminated gonococcal infection. *E. coli O157:H7* can cause a diarrheal illness with rare instances of hemolytic uremic syndrome; but the boards will give you an adequate exposure history to raw hamburger meat or petting zoos. *E. coli O157:H7* infections also usually occur in an outbreak, and several infected patients would be included in the question. *S. pneumoniae* can cause sepsis, but she has no upper respiratory symptoms; thus, this is much less likely. *N. meningitidis* is possible, but the "menses" reference implies she was possibly using tampons and, therefore, more at risk for toxic shock syndrome. If, instead, the question presented a freshman college student living in a dormitory, you should then suspect meningococcus because of the known increased risk of invasive meningococcal disease with young people living in close proximity (military or college dormitories). Finally, *S. agalactiae*, or Group B Streptococcus, is mainly a problem (especially on Board exams) of newborns, pregnant women, and diabetics.

Board Testing Point: Recognize the diagnostic criteria of toxic shock syndrome and associate the syndrome with menstruation.

195. Answer: B

Answer: *Salmonella.*
Turtle importation ceased in the 1970s; and with that, we observed a marked decrease in cases of *Salmonella* infection. However, in the 1990s and 2000s, iguanas became very popular, and there was again a big increase in the number of cases of this infection. The CDC recently reported several cases of *Salmonella* due to turtles, so be suspect of turtles on the Board examination; they are likely culprits for *Salmonella* just like our friend, the iguana. The organism is easily transmitted on fomites or from contaminated communal living areas such as the kitchen sink. Direct contact with the reservoir reptile is not required for infection. *Shigella* is not associated with reptiles. *Pasteurella* is associated with cat and dog bites, but this was not described and would be very unlikely in this clinical picture. *E. coli O157:H7* is associated with contaminated meat products or point-source outbreaks. *Carmenella* is just made up; it sounded nice and fit in with the other "ellas."

Board Testing Point: Associate *Salmonella* infection with exposures to reptiles.

196. Answer: B

Answer: *P. ovale* and *P. vivax*.
These 2 species of malaria form hypnozoites in the liver and require primaquine for effective eradication. An easy way to remember this is to associate vivax and ovale with Seagram's VO Vodka. We all know that too much vodka goes to the liver!

Board Testing Point: Synthesize treatment for malarial infections with *P. ovale* and *P. vivax*, which require primaquine to eradicate liver hypnozoites.

197. Answer: C

Answer: *Yersinia pestis*.
Of the agents listed, only *Yersinia pestis* (plague) is transferred easily from person to person in the "pneumonic" form. Bubonic plague (infection localized to the lymph nodes) is not transmissible person to person, but when the organisms spread through bacteremia to the lungs, the infection becomes markedly contagious. In this case, both men visited an area where plague is known to be endemic in the United States and may have acquired the organism through flea bites or aerosol exposure to infected animal fluids. Physicians must maintain a high index of suspicion for plague pneumonia because the organism is resistant to cephalosporins, and the infection is rapidly progressive and fatal. Additionally, because of the contagiousness of the pneumonic form, respiratory isolation must be employed early. Both anthrax and tularemia have pneumonic forms, but neither infection is transmitted person to person. Neither botulism nor *Salmonella* causes pneumonia. Remember this for the Boards: Pneumonic anthrax and tularemia do not require any special precautions; plague pneumonia definitely requires respiratory isolation!

Board Testing Point: Identify person-to-person transmission in a case of pneumonic plague.

198. Answer: E

Answer: Polymerase chain reaction (PCR) testing of CSF.
PCR testing is most likely to be positive 3 days after infection, so an initial negative PCR should be repeated at 3 days if HSV is strongly suspected. The sensitivity is between 90-98%, with a specificity of 94-100% during active infection. MRI has less sensitivity at 89% and, when abnormal, will show lesions in the temporal lobes. EEG has a sensitivity of approximately 80%, and CT scan has a sensitivity of about 55%. A viral culture of CSF is rarely positive. It used to be that the "gold standard" was brain biopsy; this has been replaced by PCR.

Board Testing Point: Recognize that CSF PCR for HSV is the most sensitive test to diagnose HSV meningoencephalitis.

199. Answer: D

Answer: Ticarcillin-clavulanic acid.
The most likely etiologic agent for the infection is *Pseudomonas*. You are given the classic history of a "nail through the tennis shoe." *Pseudomonas* is known to colonize the glue used to adhere leather in tennis shoes. Ciprofloxacin would work fine, but the patient is only 17. This drug is not approved for those under the age of 18

except as second-line therapy for UTIs and STDs. Trimethoprim-sulfamethoxazole, nafcillin, and tetracycline do not cover *Pseudomonas*.

Board Testing Point: Associate puncture injuries through tennis shoes with deep-tissue *Pseudomonas* infections; prescribe an anti-pseudomonal antibiotic appropriate for use in a 17-year-old.

200. Answer: A5, B6, C1, D3, E8, F2, G7, H4

Answers: A5, B6, C1, D3, E8, F2, G7, H4.

Board Testing Point: Associate epidemiologic specifics with respective infectious diseases.

201. Answer: C

Answer: Adenovirus.
If you selected *Mycobacterium marinum,* you could be forgiven because "swimming pool" was in the question. But there is no mention of a skin lesion. Be careful when the Board question gives you an epidemiologic clue such as geography or a specific location (like "swimming pool"), because several organisms might be associated with that clue. In this case, conjunctivitis with an epidemic-like outbreak associated with swimming pools is due to adenovirus. These outbreaks are most common in the summer; hence, the association with swimming pools. Other examples of important epidemiologic information: Arkansas + lymph node = tularemia; Arkansas + pancytopenia = ehrlichiosis; Arkansas + pneumonia + skin lesions = blastomycosis. So read the whole question and pay attention to the presentation of the infection before you jump to the most likely infection associated with the epidemiologic clue!

Board Testing Point: Recognize the association of adenovirus with swimming pools and conjunctivitis.

202. Answer: E

Answer: No additional testing is recommended.
This is very important! Physicians are commonly ordering tests for Lyme disease inappropriately, so this has become a very, very common subject for Medicine Boards. If a patient presents with only "fatigue," never order Lyme testing of any kind. The Infectious Diseases Society of America's clinical guidelines for diagnosis of Lyme disease requires 1) a disease consistent with Lyme disease (not including erythema migrans or fatigue!) and 2) exposure to a Lyme-endemic area. At this time, Texas is not a Lyme-endemic area. And to warrant further testing, she should have something else to make you think of Lyme arthritis, Bell's palsy, or carditis. A nonspecific symptom like "fatigue" does not warrant an investigation for Lyme.

To clarify, the classic erythema migrans rash of Lyme is so characteristic that if you see it, and the history is appropriate for exposure to possible Lyme, go ahead and treat as though the rash is due to Lyme. Serology is frequently not positive at the time of the rash. Additionally, serology is not very good, and false positives are common. Polymerase chain reaction has only been useful in cases of Lyme arthritis, and positive results are not consistent. In cases of known Lyme meningitis, PCR testing has been negative. Hence, PCR testing is not recommended except in rare cases of Lyme arthritis. Check Lyme serology only in a patient who has clinical criteria for Lyme and has been in a Lyme-prone area!

Board Testing Point: Identify appropriate situations for Lyme testing.

203. Answer: C

Answer: Parvovirus B-19.
It appears that the niece had fifth's disease, which is caused by parvovirus B-19. This can be diagnosed by the historical description of the classic facial rash. In adults exposed to this virus who do not already have immunity, it is not unusual to develop arthritis of the smaller joints, particularly in the hands, and a reticular rash. To confirm the diagnosis, check parvovirus B-19 IgM antibodies. PCR is available to confirm intrauterine infections using amniotic fluid. Only Still's disease looks somewhat akin to a parvo infection, but very elevated ferritin levels (> 50,000) is more consistent with Still's disease, and the rash typically appears only during periods of fever. Rheumatoid arthritis would not present with these joint manifestations. Coxsackievirus and echovirus do not normally cause arthritis symptoms.

Board Testing Point: Recognize the association of small joint arthritis and exposure to children with parvovirus B-19.

204. Answer: B

Answer: Nafcillin.
With her history of influenza, she is at high risk for a secondary bacterial infection, specifically pneumonia, from pneumococcus or *Staphylococcus aureus*. Her blood culture, however, suggests *S. aureus* given the "grape-clustered" morphology; *S. pneumoniae* would have diplococcal morphology. Of the options listed, nafcillin is the more directed therapy. Piperacillin/tazobactam would also be effective, but is much too broad in spectrum. IV ceftriaxone is not appropriate since it lacks coverage for *S. aureus*. IV trimethoprim-sulfamethoxazole is not a good choice for this infection but would be the drug of choice if *Pneumocystis* were a concern. Finally, oral amoxicillin/clavulanic acid is not appropriate for bacteremia. This antibiotic would be fine for a localized skin infection but not a serious life-threatening pneumonia or bacteremia.

Board Testing Point: Associate *S. aureus* as an etiology of the secondary bacterial pneumonia of influenza.

205. Answer: E

Answer: No further immunizations at this time.
Here are the guidelines to remember:

Wound is <u>dirty</u> and either patient has
      1. < 3 immunizations, OR
      2. Immunization history unknown = Give TIG + vaccine

Wound is <u>clean</u> and immunizations are up-to-date (i.e. is has been < 10 years since last immunization) = No Treatment

Wound is <u>dirty</u> and immunizations are up to date, with most recent < 5 years = No Treatment

So this woman has a dirty wound and had a booster Td < 5 years ago; therefore, she is protected and does not need further immunizations at this time.

Board Testing Point: Interpret guidelines for tetanus immunization in adults.

206. Answer: B

Answer: *Clostridium botulinum*.
Botulism is mediated by a toxin generated by *C. botulinum* under anaerobic conditions. The toxin is heat labile, but may not be inactivated under standard cooking conditions. The classic presentation of botulism is a descending paralysis with involvement of extraocular and pharyngeal muscles progressing to respiratory compromise. Sensory function is unaffected, but the patient may experience confusion. Risk for botulism includes foods that are prepared in home bottling and preservation techniques that allow propagation of the botulism organism or fail to destroy formed toxin. Some traditional foods of various ethnic groups meet these criteria.

Bacillus cereus usually presents with abdominal pain and diarrhea, but uncommonly produces a neurotoxin that results in a significant element of vomiting. Enterotoxigenic *E. coli* results in watery diarrhea without a direct neurological involvement. Shigella species may produce a variety of symptoms based on the various organism types. Patients may have diarrhea and increased fever, which in younger and susceptible individuals may result in seizure activity. Neurologic manifestations also include seizures associated with hyponatremia and hypoglycemia. Less common is encephalopathy, which presents with unusual posturing and cerebral edema. Descending paralysis is not part of the shigella constellation of symptoms.

Board Testing Point: Recognize the findings of botulism.

207. Answer: B

Answer: Diagnosis of acute rheumatic fever in an adult presenting with migratory arthritis and a new heart murmur requires confirmatory evidence of recent Group A streptococcal infection.
Pharyngeal strains of Group A streptococcus (GAS) are responsible for rheumatic fever, not the skin or soft tissue strains. Prophylactic antibiotics are necessary for at least 5 years for all patients with rheumatic fever, regardless of the presence or absence of carditis. Acute rheumatic fever occurs remotely to the pharyngeal infection--which is why you can delay therapy for GAS infection pending throat culture results. Delaying therapy for a few days will not increase the risk of rheumatic fever.

Board Testing Point: Recognize the presentation of acute rheumatic fever and offer adequate counseling on pathogenesis.

208. Answer: E

Answer: No treatment is recommended.
A urine exposure to intact skin requires no post-exposure prophylaxis. If this had been a needle-stick, then starting HAART (highly active anti-retroviral therapy) with AZT + 3TC (Combivir®) and indinavir (Crixivan®) would have been correct. Use of genotype testing has not been evaluated and currently is not recommended by the CDC. Using a single drug is never the correct answer. Using 2 drugs is appropriate in some circumstances, but the Boards will usually ask you a straightforward "no therapy" or 3-drug therapy question for post-exposure prophylaxis.

Board Testing Point: Synthesize a post-exposure prophylaxis regimen after various HIV exposures.

209. Answer: D

Answer: IV vancomycin and IV ceftriaxone.
The scenario doesn't give us much information, but you must assume that the two most likely organisms are *Streptococcus pneumoniae* and *Neisseria meningitidis.* For *Neisseria,* ampicillin or ceftriaxone is likely adequate; but for *S. pneumoniae,* vancomycin should be added initially until you know the sensitivities for the organism. The clues that she works in a daycare center and had a recent cold should raise your suspicions that she has been exposed to resistant pneumococci, because infants and children in daycare settings are more likely to be colonized or infected with penicillin-resistant pneumonococcus. Be aware also that in some parts of the U.S., 8-10% of *S. pneumoniae* are resistant to ceftriaxone.

Board Testing Point: Prescribe the appropriate empiric regimen for meningitis by synthesizing the most probable bacterial etiologies: *Neisseria* and penicillin-resistant *Streptococcus pneumoniae.*

210. Answer: C

Answer: *E. coli.*
In men over the age of 35, *E. coli* is the most common cause of epididymitis. Even if you suspect that he isn't monogamous, *E. coli* is still #1 in his age group. If he were in his 20s, then *Chlamydia trachomatis* would be the most likely. *Neisseria* rarely causes epididymitis compared to *Chlamydia,* and *Pseudomonas* almost never is implicated.

Board Testing Point: Estimate the most common organism causing epididymitis in those over 35 years of age.

211. Answer: D

Answer: Benzathine penicillin G 2.4 million units IM.
For primary syphilis and secondary syphilis (< 1 year since acquiring the infection), one dose of long-acting penicillin is appropriate. Procaine penicillin should not be prescribed unless it is combined with probenecid to prolong the half-life of penicillin. Ceftriaxone is not recommended by the CDC for primary syphilis. If he was penicillin-allergic, you would prescribe doxycycline 100 mg bid x 14 days.

Board Testing Point: Recognize that a chancre classifies a patient like this as having primary syphilis and prescribe the appropriate treatment for this stage.

212. Answer: C

Answer: Doxycycline.
Mycoplasma or *Chlamydophila pneumoniae* (formerly *Chlamydia pneumoniae* or TWAR) is the most likely etiology of pneumonia in an adolescent who is not that ill. Of the choices, doxycycline and levofloxacin would cover these 2 organisms well (amoxicillin, ceftriaxone, and trimethoprim-sulfamethoxazole have virtually no coverage). It is possible he has pneumococcus, but that is less likely with his symptoms. Luckily, doxycycline would cover pneumococcus as well. What is wrong with levofloxacin? Too expensive! Yes, compared to doxycycline, but the real reason is his age: he is under 18! Azithromycin or erythromycin would also be acceptable answers.

Testing Point: Identify and treat the most common etiologies of community-acquired pneumonia *(Mycoplasma* and *Chlamydophila)* in adolescents and young adults.

213. Answer: D

Answer: Meningococcemia.
This patient is presenting with fever and a rapidly progressive painful acral rash in association with hypotension and disseminated intravascular coagulopathy (DIC), which is consistent with purpura fulminans. Meningococcemia is the most common cause of purpura fulminans and commonly leads to early septic shock and organ dysfunction. Although secondary syphilis causes an acral rash, it is not associated with coagulopathy; and the lesions are maculopapular, not petechial/purpuric. Toxic shock syndrome certainly causes shock, multiple organ injury, and DIC; but, the rash is a diffuse blanching erythema. Rocky Mountain Spotted Fever does cause an acral petechial rash and the patient has had exposure to dog ticks, but DIC is uncommon (< 10%), and the infection is rare after September in the calendar year. Also, the incubation period is usually > 3 days, and the rash typically occurs > 5d after the onset of fever. Gonococcemia rarely causes organ failure or DIC, and the rash is usually a smattering of pustules.

Board Testing Point: Recognize the presentation of meningococcemia.

214. Answer: A

Answer: HBsAG: Negative; HBcAg: Positive; Anti-HBsAg: Positive. Remote infection has resolved.
Option B is immunization.
Option C is either active or chronic infection.
Option D is no infection and no immunization.
Option E is either more than one infection or chronic infection with immunization.

Board Testing Point: Interpret hepatitis serology

215. Answer: C

Answer: Vancomycin, tobramycin, and ceftazidime.
He is quite ill-appearing and definitely has infection (fever, increased purulent sputum production), so "no therapy" is not correct. They tell you that he has had MRSA and various *Pseudomonas* infections in the past (presence of these organisms from a bronchoscopy specimen implicates them as pathogens as opposed to simply colonizers of the upper airways). With his current probable pneumonia, you have to suspect that he is infected with either or both of these. Therefore, you need to include coverage for both in your empiric regimen. Vancomycin, remember, is the only antibiotic listed effective against serious MRSA, so it is required in the regimen. That leaves us with vancomycin + ceftriaxone + tobramycin and vancomycin + tobramycin + ceftazidime. Ceftriaxone is ineffective against *Pseudomonas*; therefore, the only choice here is vancomycin, tobramycin, and ceftazidime. Aminoglycosides are the drugs of choice for serious pseudomonas infections.

Board Testing Point: Interpret bronchoscopy cultures and design a treatment regimen for a patient with a cystic fibrosis exacerbation.

216. Answer: A

Answer: *Ehrlichia*.
This patient has typical ehrlichiosis. If you see the words "Arkansas," "tick bite," and "pancytopenia," think ehrlichiosis due to *Ehrlichia chaffeensis*. The bone marrow is showing the classic "morula" of *Ehrlichia*, which also can be seen in a peripheral smear sometimes. Of course, RMSF is endemic to the same area, but these

patients in the Board exams will have petechial rashes around their wrists and ankles, and they will be much more ill. Other potential clinical manifestations often included in patient scenarios include hyponatremia and elevated LFTs. Both RMSF and *Ehrlichia* present with the pancytopenia (and possibly the sodium and LFT derangements, as well.) While *Ehrlichia* doesn't classically have a rash, and is called "Rocky Mountain Spotless Fever," it is not uncommon to see a mild diffuse erythematous rash on the trunk. But, you do not see the RMSF petechial rash. Various forms of *Ehrlichia* are seen also in Missouri, Wisconsin, and the Northeast. He does not live in a Lyme-endemic area or a plague area (*Yersinia*). *Francisella* would cause an enlarged lymph node with or without an ulcerated lesion and does not cause pancytopenia. *Klebsiella* does not cause this sort of clinical presentation.

Board Testing Point: Identify ehrlichiosis based on epidemiologic clues, clinical history, and laboratory testing.

217. Answer: B

Answer: *Bacillus anthracis*.
Of the agents listed, anthrax (*B. anthracis*) will cause pneumonia with a widened mediastinum and, importantly, is not spread person to person via the respiratory route, as are plague (*Y. pestis*) and smallpox. Smallpox pneumonia would be rare and would not present with a widened mediastinum. Plague would present as a hemorrhagic pneumonia. Human herpesvirus 6 causes roseola, a common childhood illness that would not cause pneumonia.

Board Testing Point: Differentiate between plague and anthrax pneumonia based on clinical findings.

218. Answer: C

Answer: The anesthesiologist who intubated the patient.
The medical student and resident did not have close exposure to upper respiratory secretions where meningococci colonize the nasopharynx. Since there is a possibility that the anesthesiologist did get exposed to secretions when intubating the patient, s/he is the only one who should be offered prophylaxis.

Board Testing Point: Determine who should receive meningococcal prophylaxis.

219. Answer: A

Answer: Reassurance that the findings are normal.
During testicular self exam or following a course in sex education, males will often present with concern that they have a sexually transmitted disease. The findings described above are typical for pearly penile papules, a normal finding in 15-20% of pubertal and postpubertal males. They are differentiated from genital warts in that the size of the papules is similar and their appearance does not change over time. Herpetic lesions are typically tender and grouped. Syphilitic lesions present as small painless ulcers. Dysuria, frequency and penile discharge suggest infection with *Chlamydia* and/or Gonorrhea.

Board Testing Point: Recognize that pearly penile papules are common and should not be confused with genital warts or other STD-like lesions.

220. Answer: C

Answer: Obtain a heterophile antibody test.
The patient most likely has infectious mononucleosis. The heterophile antibody test is a qualitative rapid slide test using horse erythrocytes. It detects heterophile antibody in > 90% of adolescents and adults with mononucleosis. A majority of patients with infectious mononucleosis develop a rash with amoxicillin. Hepatomegaly is seen in 10-15% of patients with mononucleosis. His symptoms are not consistent with Rocky Mountain Spotted Fever. A throat culture for Group A Streptococcus at this point is unnecessary since he developed a rash while being treated with amoxicillin. This rash is so specific to these circumstances that a patient who develops it in the context of a mono-like illness should be assumed to have mononucleosis. An investigation for EBV-associated mono should be performed now. Erythromycin will be no more effective in treating this virus than amoxicillin. Hepatitis would not present with pharyngitis, and rickettsial presentation would almost always offer clues of tick-bite or geography to help you.

Board Testing Point: Recognize that a misdiagnosed Group A Streptococcal infection is most likely to be infectious mononucleosis, and that such patients treated with amoxicillin will develop a rash.

221. Answer: A

Answer: Crowded living conditions increase the risk of disease.
This is a case of fulminant meningococcemia. Definitive diagnosis requires culture of the organism from the blood or cerebral spinal fluid, but Gram stain of petechial/purpuric lesions may be positive for the organism (note the intracellular Gram-negative diplococci seen on his Gram stain). College students, especially those living in dormitory settings or other crowded conditions, are at increased risk, along with children < 2 years of age. Both the polysaccharide and newer conjugate vaccines provide coverage for meningococcal groups A, C, Y and W135, but not group B. The disease is primarily spread by respiratory droplet. The most common neurologic sequela is hearing loss in 5-15% of individuals surviving the disease.

Board Testing Point: Know that meningococcal disease is much more common in college students and those living in closely confined areas.

NEPHROLOGY

222. Answer: B

Answer: Refer to a urologist for cystoscopy.
This is a case of iron deficiency anemia, as determined through analysis of a % saturation that is < 20 and a low serum ferritin. Iron deficiency is never normal in an adult male, and though iron supplements may be required, a diagnosis as to the etiology of blood loss should be sought. Guaiac studies alone are insufficient to dismiss a GI source, and this patient may benefit from evaluation of the colon. His acute evaluation, however, has identified a potential renal source. Ultrasound and abdominal CT can help identify renal masses and structural abnormalities but do not effectively visualize the bladder for malignancies or lesions. Cystoscopy is required. This patient has normal initial prostate studies, so random biopsy is not indicated. Infection is the most common cause of urinary bleeding, but the patient demonstrates no evidence of an active infectious process, and there is no significant pyuria. The blood counts and iron studies are consistent with iron deficiency, and bone marrow is not necessary to evaluate either iron stores or hematopoietic capacity.

Board Testing Point: Refer a patient who presents with iron-deficiency anemia and microscopic hematuria for cystoscopy.

223. Answer: A

Answer: Stress incontinence.
Stress incontinence occurs when the urinary sphincter is unable to prevent spontaneous passage of urine when abdominal pressure is increased. This can occur with laughing, coughing, or sudden jars to the body. Neurogenic bladder arises from difficulty with detrusor muscle function that prevents complete urine emptying with normal voids and results in urinary retention and overflow incontinence. Urge incontinence presents with an urgent need to urinate and little ability to suppress spontaneous contraction of the bladder. Patients with normal bladder function, but who have difficulty meeting the physical demands of voiding, may experience functional incontinence. This includes patients with diseases such as Parkinson disease, severe arthritis, or general weakness.

Board Testing Point: Discuss and define causes of urinary abnormalities in a post-menopausal woman.

224. Answer: D

Answer: Cystoscopy.
Interstitial cystitis is a chronic inflammatory condition affecting the bladder. The reasons for the inflammation remain under investigation, and an active infectious agent has not been implicated. The inflammation produces fibrosis of the wall of the bladder that limits its capacity to expand and causes symptoms when urine stretches the restricted bladder. The normal adult bladder volume is typically 400-500 cc., but this patient's is reduced to 250 cc. At this smaller capacity, the patient experiences the sensation of bladder fullness and requires more frequent urination. Interstitial cystitis is best diagnosed by cystoscopy. IVP, renal US, and pelvic CT do not adequately demonstrate this condition.

Board Testing Point: Specify the findings and workup of intersitial cystitis.

225. Answer: A

Answer: Volume repletion with IV crystalloid.
A key point in the management of hyperkalemia is that hemodialysis is indicated following the appropriate trial of medical management. Given the hemodynamics and a clinical situation where you suspect that the patient is intravascularly (or effectively intravascularly) volume-depleted, IV crystalloid as a volume resuscitation is the first step. If his limited urine output is at all related to his volume depletion, increasing tubular flow with delivery of sodium to the distal nephron will be essential in the excretion of potassium. While IV insulin/glucose and Kayexalate will each lower serum potassium levels, they are not the best initial management treatments in this patient given his hemodynamics. Calcium gluconate does not have a role in therapy at this point, but would be reserved if ECG changes were occurring.

Board Testing Point: Manage hyperkalemia and identify when to initiate dialysis.

226. Answer: B

Answer: Urate stone.
This patient's clinical presentation is consistent with nephrolithiasis. A stone that is not seen on KUB but is demonstrated on ultrasound is consistent with a radiolucent kidney stone. Cysteine stones contain significant amounts of sulfur, which is thought to make them visible on x-ray studies. Struvite is typically composed of calcium- and magnesium-containing substances that also make them radio-opaque. The calcium in the calcium oxalate and calcium phosphate make these stones highly visible on radiological studies. Urate stones are radiolucent, which is consistent with this scenario and the picture is showing a uric acid crystal. A patient with renal papillary necrosis and a sloughed papilla in the ureter may also present with similar findings.

Board Testing Point: Distinguish the radiolucency of various kidney stones.

227. Answer: D

Answer: One ampule of IV calcium gluconate.
Hyperkalemia in the setting of ECG changes indicates a risk for prolongation of the QRS complex, resulting in ventricular tachycardia. He has peaked T-waves as well as widening of his QRS complexes. IV insulin/glucose and Kayexalate® will both lower serum potassium, but stabilization of the membrane of cardiac cells is **essential** to prevent arrhythmias, so the most appropriate next step is administration of IV calcium gluconate. Volume repletion and sodium polystyrene sulfonate infusion can be used as adjuncts but are not the best answer for severe hyperkalemia resulting in ECG changes.

Board Testing Point: Manage hyperkalemia in the face of peaked T waves after volume repletion.

228. Answer: D

Answer: Pericarditis secondary to uremia.
Given her small size and advanced age, a creatinine of 1.8 represents severe loss of kidney function. While a pulmonary embolism is possible given her past medical history, her A-a gradient is 14 (normal for her age is < 23) making an acute PE unlikely. Evaluation of her acid/base status reveals an elevated anion gap acidosis, and an obvious etiology of elevated anions in this clinical scenario includes the anions of renal failure. Her electrocardiogram demonstrates diffuse ST elevation and is more consistent with pericarditis than ischemia. Pericardial fluid in uremic pericarditis is usually bland, but can undergo hemorrhagic transformation when

inadvertently treated with anticoagulants or antiplatelet drugs. Empiric treatment with drugs that impair clotting should not be performed when pericarditis is in the differential diagnosis until pericarditis can be definitively excluded.

Board Testing Point: Deduce from studies and history that pericarditis is a reason to initiate dialysis.

229. Answer: A

Answer: Specific gravity: 1.010, pH: 7.0, protein: neg, blood: neg, microscopic exam: coarse granular casts.
This urine is classic for a more general appearance of acute tubular necrosis, perhaps related to hypotension. Of note, the specific gravity is isosthenuric and pH is more neutral, indicating limited tubular function. Granular casts are indicative of tubular damage.

Board Testing Point: Compare and contrast various urinalysis findings, and identify tubular necrosis.

230. Answer: D

Answer: Specific gravity: 1.020, pH: 5.5, protein: neg, blood: neg, microscopic exam: calcium oxalate crystals.
Ethylene glycol ingestion is associated with an increased amount of calcium oxalate in the urine. The appearance of these "coffin-lid" crystals can provide a key diagnostic clue toward the presence of this ingestion.

Board Testing Point: Compare and contrast various urinalysis findings, and identify ingestion of ethylene glycol.

231. Answer: A

Answer: Urine color: red, blood by dipstick of urine: present, microscopic exam: no RBCs, color of plasma: red.
Differentiating these urinalyses requires consideration of the dipstick results, the microscopic exam, and the color of plasma. Free hemoglobin in plasma will result in the color of plasma being red. This is the difference between hemoglobinuria and myoglobinuria. Of note, they both will have a strongly positive urine dipstick for blood, but no RBCs present on microscopic exam. Individual medications may turn the urine different colors (rifampin = orange, phenazopyridine = orange, Aldomet® = black, phenolphthalein = red). Clearly in these circumstances, you would not expect dipstick or microscopic exam of the urine to indicate blood.

Board Testing Point: Interpret urinalyses, and identify hemoglobinuria.

232. Answer: B

Answer: Urine color: red, blood by dipstick of urine: present, microscopic exam: no RBCs, color of plasma: clear.
Differentiating these urinalyses requires consideration of the dipstick results, the microscopic exam, and the color of plasma. Free hemoglobin in plasma will result in the color of plasma being red. This is the difference between hemoglobinuria and myoglobinuria. Of note, they both will have a strongly positive urine dipstick for blood, but no RBCs present on microscopic exam. Individual medications may turn the urine different colors (rifampin = orange, phenazopyridine = orange, Aldomet® = black, phenolphthalein = red). Clearly in these circumstances, you would not expect dipstick or microscopic exam of the urine to indicate blood.

Board Testing Point: Interpret urinalyses, and identify myoglobinuria.

233. Answer: D

Answer: Urine color: red, blood by dipstick of urine: absent, microscopic exam: no RBCs, color of plasma: clear.
Differentiating these urinalyses requires consideration of the dipstick results, the microscopic exam, and the color of plasma. Free hemoglobin in plasma will result in the color of plasma being red. This is the difference between hemoglobinuria and myoglobinuria. Of note, they both will have a strongly positive urine dipstick for blood, but no RBCs present on microscopic exam. Individual medications may turn the urine different colors (rifampin = orange, phenazopyridine = orange, Aldomet® = black, phenolphthalein = red). Clearly in these circumstances, you would not expect dipstick or microscopic exam of the urine to indicate blood.

Board Testing Point: To be able to interpret urinalyses, and identify phenolphthalein.

234. Answer: B

Answer: Renal biopsy.
Given this patient's age and race, the most likely idiopathic glomerular lesion would be membranous nephropathy. Renal biopsy would be essential toward making that diagnosis. Of note: while he is diabetic, the time course of his diabetes relative to his presentation with glomerular disease is not consistent with his diabetes playing a role in his nephropathy. Among patients with type 1 DM, nephropathy is usually diagnosed after 10-15 years since onset. Due to the more incipient initiation of diabetes among patients with type 2 DM, the onset of proteinuria is much shorter at 3-5 years after diagnosis of DM. For this reason, an ophthalmologic exam to evaluate for diabetic retinopathy is not likely to provide diagnostic clues. Empiric therapy with an ACE-I is not unreasonable for any glomerular disease, but the sudden onset of nephrotic range proteinuria is deserving of a kidney biopsy. You would want renal tissue first before using steroids to see if it might be steroid responsive. A tagged WBC scan would be of no clinical use in this scenario.

Board Testing Point: Determine when renal biopsy is indicated in the presence of specific symptoms and studies.

235. Answer: A

Answer: Anti-DNAse B.
Based on the presence of RBC casts and glomerular damage in the urine, this patient has acute glomerulonephritis that is likely rapidly progressive. Goodpasture disease has a bimodal distribution in terms of age and could be a possibility in a man in his 70s. Anti-GBM antibody could be measured but is not a choice here. Similarly, Wegner granulomatosis could be a possibility and would be assessed using ANCA testing. However, we have provided evidence of an antecedent streptococcal infection: the occurrence of a post-CABG, rapidly progressive, erythematous soft tissue infection with raised borders in the setting of tinea pedis is suggestive of erysipelas from Group A streptococci. Given this, post-streptococcal glomerulonephritis is the most likely etiology of his renal failure with an active sediment. Note also that post-streptococcal glomerulonephritis can occur approximately two weeks following pharyngitis and is marked by elevated ASO titers. However, the presentation may be three weeks later following skin infection, and the anti-DNAse B is more likely to be positive in this setting. ESR and C-reactive protein are nonspecific tests. Hemoglobin A1C, although helpful for determining diabetes control, would not be helpful in diagnosing post-streptococcal disease.

Board Testing Point: Reconstruct the findings in post-streptococcal glomerulonephritis.

236. Answer: C

Answer: Anticoagulation with heparin.
In this patient presenting with acute flank pain, one must consider the possibility of nephrolithiasis and pyelonephritis. Diagnostic evaluation should include a spiral CT and an ultrasound; but in the face of fever and leukocytosis, infection must also be considered. What is important about this patient is that he has atrial fibrillation, is not already on anticoagulation, and has acute flank pain. This patient most likely had a clot embolize to the right renal artery. LDH is markedly elevated in renal infarction, and may be very helpful in this clinical situation. Once suspected, diagnostic evaluation that assesses renal flow is essential, and the patient must be immediately anticoagulated.

Board Testing Point: Evaluate acute right flank pain and associate systemic embolization to the kidney as a sequela of atrial fibrillation.

237. Answer: B

Answer: Takayasu arteritis.
The sudden onset of hypertension, particularly in younger women, should raise the possibility of renal artery stenosis. The most common etiology of renal artery stenosis in this age group is fibromuscular dysplasia, which can cause unilateral renal artery stenosis, and is usually amenable to angioplasty. However, in a patient with constitutional symptoms, a systemic disease (such as a vasculitis) should be considered. The vasculitis most likely to cause renal artery stenosis in women of this age group is Takayasu arteritis. This large vessel vasculitis may cause symptoms of claudication in the upper extremities, as well as renal artery disease. Polyarteritis nodosa and polymyalgia rheumatica would be seen in much older individuals.

Board Testing Point: Associate Takayasu arteritis and renal artery stenosis.

238. Answer: C

Answer: The risk of the procedure will be significantly lower if he is hydrated with normal saline before and after the angiography.
The decision to proceed with any procedure is based on the risk-to-benefit ratio. Reducing the risk of radiocontrast dye-induced acute renal failure has been the subject of significant evaluation over the last several years, particularly in at-risk patients. Greater risk is associated with Class III or IV heart failure, diabetes, serum creatinine > 1.6 mg/dL, age > 75 years, larger volumes of contrast material, shock, and anemia. Data are most consistent in demonstrating a reduced risk of contrast-induced nephropathy when .9% saline is administered for 24 h prior to the procedure. Risk may also be reduced by using low osmolality contrast agents. Initial studies have supported the use of either sodium bicarbonate or n-acetylcysteine as prophylactic agents. However, either the numbers of studies have been limited or meta-analyses have been inconclusive and further investigation is warranted. Both diuretics and non-steroidal anti-inflammatory drugs should be withheld for 24 hours prior to the study, and metformin should be withheld for at least 48 hours. Candesartan has not been shown to be a factor, and using furosemide beforehand would actually worsen hydration.

Board Testing Point: Modify the risk of dye-induced renal toxicity by hydration.

239. Answer: C

Answer: Hydrochlorothiazide.
This patient has Gordon syndrome, a rare inherited tubular disorder in which there is increased fractional proximal reabsorption of sodium, decreased mineralocorticoid activity, and suppression of aldosterone but a normal GFR. Renin activity is suppressed. This is a heterogeneous genetic disorder with abnormalities that have been described on chromosome 1, 17, and 12. Mutations have been described in the WNK family of serine threonine kinases that localize to the distal nephron. Thiazide diuretics inhibit sodium resorption in the distal tubule mediated by ENaC (the electroneutral Na/Cl cotransporter). Na resorption is then increased in the cortical collecting duct, which increases K and H secretion. Treatment with Kayexalate® would lower potassium, but will not treat the underlying disorder. The electrolytes are also typical of Type IV RTA; however, these patients can increase their aldosterone levels and are typically diabetic. Gordon syndrome is one type of pseudohypoaldosteronism. Indomethacin would be completely inappropriate and would exacerbate the hyperkalemia by increasing proximal sodium reabsorption and suppressing aldosterone. Sulfinpyrazone and fludrocortisone have no role in treatment.

Board Testing Point: Interpret laboratories and diagnose/treat Gordon syndrome.

240. Answer: D

Answer: Propylene glycol toxicity.
This patient has an anion gap metabolic acidosis, excluding the possibility of an RTA. Patients with sepsis most commonly will have a lactic acidosis. No clinical evidence points to sepsis, despite the high risk in patients with extensive burns. Patients with starvation ketosis have a mild anion gap acidosis, typically with ketones in the urine. Both lysine and arginine may lead to a non-anion gap metabolic acidosis, typically occurring in patients receiving IV hyperalimentation. Propylene glycol is a vehicle that is contained in sulfadiazine and several intravenous medications, such as nitroglycerin, diazepam, and lorazepam. It is metabolized to lactic acid by hepatic alcohol dehydrogenase and may potentially cause an anion gap metabolic acidosis.

Board Testing Point: Evaluate potential causes of anion gap metabolic acidosis.

241. Answer: E

Answer: Hydrochlorothiazide 25 mg daily.
This patient's presentation is typical for recurrent nephrolithiasis. She was appropriately evaluated at least 6 weeks after resolution of an acute episode. The most common identifiable cause is hypercalciuria, defined as more than 4 mg/kg/day. While the weight is not provided for this patient, it is clearly elevated. All patients with stone disease should increase their fluid intake to at least 2 L per day. Treatment of hypercalciuria includes reducing protein and sodium intake, as well as thiazide therapy in doses from 25-100 mg/d. It is not necessary to discontinue calcium carbonate therapy in patients with hypercalciuria, unless one can demonstrate that discontinuing the dose reduces urinary excretion of calcium. Allopurinol therapy is appropriate for patients with hyperuricosuria or patients with calcium stones with a uric acid nidus. Alkalinization is also helpful for patients with uric acid stones, either with bicarbonate solutions or, if inadequate, with acetazolamide. There may also be a benefit to increasing the urinary pH in cystinuria, but additional therapy with tiopronin or penicillamine is usually necessary.

Board Testing Point: Prescribe treatment for hypercalciuria.

242. Answer: D

Answer: Nuclear polyoma virus inclusions.
The most likely diagnosis in this patient is allograft nephropathy secondary to BK virus, one of the polyoma viruses. Diagnosis can be suspected by the identification of virus inclusion-bearing cells in the urine (decoy cells), which are present in about 30% of affected patients. Confirmation requires renal biopsy. When focal segmental glomerulosclerosis (FSGS) recurs, it typically does so in the immediate post-transplant period and is associated with proteinuria. The time period for acute cellular rejection is appropriate in this patient and would definitely be part of the differential diagnosis. While proteinuria might suggest this diagnosis, often the only abnormality is seen on renal biopsy. Tacrolimus toxicity is dose-dependent and can occur in patients with normal tacrolimus levels, and confirmed if renal function improves when the dose is lowered. Usually, however, levels are clearly elevated or are in the upper end of the therapeutic range. Clues to the diagnosis of CMV infection include fever, leukopenia, and abnormalities of liver function tests. Diagnosis is usually established by DNA quantitation by PCR.

Board Testing Point: Evaluate etiologies of post-transplant rejection.

243. Answer: B

Answer: Type II RTA.
First, recognize this is a case of hypokalemia and second, this is a patient with a non-anion gap hyperchloremic metabolic acidosis (138-[114 + 20] = Anion gap = 4 or if you like to include the K the anion gap is 6.8, which is still normal). In this case, differential diagnosis excludes Bartter syndrome as it causes a metabolic alkalosis. Type IV RTA is a hyperkalemic form of RTA, and therefore, is also excluded. (Consider this memory trick: "Type IV, or 4" correlates with hyperkalemia in the sense that if a potassium level is "4", it would be normal to high and not LOW.) The urine pH is consistent with either Type I or Type II RTA; what is unique about this case is the hypophosphatemia, hypouricemia, and renal glycosuria, typical of Fanconi syndrome, which is associated with Type II RTA.

Board Testing Point: Interpret serum and urine laboratory data and diagnose Type II renal tubular acidosis.

244. Answer: A

Answer: Serum renin-0.09, serum aldosterone-205.
In this case, one must decide what values are likely to be found in a patient with a unilateral adrenal mass. In determining whether his mass is an adenoma versus a malignancy, we can consider the size of the mass, and whether or not symptoms of hormone activity are present. Malignant tumors are more likely to be larger (3-6 cm), so his tumor at 1.5 cm is considered "small" and less likely to be malignant. Because of his hypertension, hypokalemia, and metabolic alkalosis, his mass is assumed to be hormonally active; this makes malignancy unlikely. In patients who present with hypertension, hypokalemia, and a metabolic alkalosis, the two most common causes are either primary or secondary hyperaldosteronism due to renovascular disease, or primary hyperaldosteronism due to a mass lesion in the adrenal gland. Tests of choice to evaluate possible hyperaldosteronism are upright plasma renin levels (which should be suppressed by excess aldo) and plasma aldosterone levels (which are elevated). The CT scan establishes the diagnosis in this patient and is confirmed when aldosterone is elevated and renin is low. In renovascular disease, the renin and aldosterone levels are both high, while in Liddle syndrome, which can present with hypertension, hypokalemia, and metabolic alkalosis, renin and aldosterone levels are low. Liddle syndrome is extremely rare.

Board Testing Point: Interpret laboratory tests and diagnose a hormonally-active adrenal mass causing primary hyperaldosteronism.

245. Answer: C

Answer: Restrict salt and water intake to 500 cc/day.
Based on the clinical information, this patient has cirrhosis, which results in both salt and water retention; and when severe, results in hyponatremia due to simulation of ADH. In asymptomatic hyponatremic patients with sodium levels > 120 mEq/L, loose water restriction is recommended, since there is very little benefit in causing a patient to become more thirsty to raise a low laboratory value, from which the patient is asymptomatic anyway. However, as the sodium level falls below 120 mEq/L, risks for neurologic impairment increases, and these patients should be treated more aggressively. Therefore, it would be most appropriate to restrict both salt and water. In patients with symptomatic hyponatremia (mental status changes, seizures), 3% saline would be appropriate. This patient does not fit that category. One would not give either saline or water, because these would exacerbate either the hyponatremia or the ascites. One could give a diuretic if the patient does not respond to salt and water restriction, but it may worsen hypokalemia and increase the risk of hepatic encephalopathy.

Board Testing Point: Choose the best treatment for SIADH.

246. Answer: C

Answer: Administer acetazolamide.
As in all acid-base scenarios, use a stepwise approach: acidemia vs alkalemia, metabolic vs respiratory, simple vs mixed disturbance. The first thing to recognize in this scenario is that the patient is alkalemic and second, that the primary problem is a metabolic alkalosis. The next question is whether this is a simple or mixed acid-base disturbance: i.e., is the patient's respiratory response to the metabolic alkalosis physiologically appropriate? The pCO_2 should increase by .5-.7 for every 1 mEq/L increase in the serum HCO_3. In this patient the pCO_2 did not increase at all; therefore, the patient is hyperventilating and must also have a respiratory alkalosis. This is therefore a mixed metabolic and respiratory alkalosis. In cases like this, one should always calculate the anion gap to assure there is not a hidden "triple acid-base disturbance;" i.e., if the AG was high, there could be a superimposed metabolic acidosis, but that information is not provided here.

In this scenario, there are several etiologies for his metabolic alkalosis, including steroid administration, nasogastric suction, and post-hypercapnia. In light of his COPD and increased A-a gradient, he is unlikely to be taken off of steroids or extubated. Volume depletion frequently contributes to metabolic alkalosis and should be considered in all cases; however, he is unlikely to be volume-depleted because he is receiving IV fluids and his diuretic was discontinued. One can correct metabolic alkalosis with the administration of .1N HCL, which must be given through a central line; but it should be reserved for extreme cases where other forms of therapy are unlikely to be effective. Acetazolamide inhibits carbonic anhydrase in the proximal tubule and therefore causes the kidney to lose HCO_3, analogous to a Type II (proximal) RTA. Therefore, acetazolamide can be used to correct metabolic alkalosis in patients who require a diuretic, but who have other ongoing problems that make other forms of therapy difficult.

Board Testing Point: Interpret a blood gas and prescribe appropriate therapy for the acid/base disturbance.

247. Answer: A

Answer: Na 115, K 3.2, Cl 72, CO$_2$ 31, BUN 45, Cr 1.6, Glu 101, pH 7.47, Urine Na 11.
There is a metabolic alkalosis, pre-renal azotemia, and the patient is trying to avidly retain sodium. This would be expected in either a volume-depleted patient who had been vomiting, or had been taking diuretics but stopped. If the patient was still on diuretics, the urine sodium would still be high. If the patient was still vomiting, he would be losing bicarbonate in the urine, which would cause urinary sodium losses, despite volume contraction, because bicarbonate acts as a non-resorbable anion in the tubule and takes sodium with it. In this case, one could measure urinary chloride, which would be low, and is therefore helpful in assessing metabolic alkalosis.

Board Testing Point: Evaluate electrolytes and urine sodiums with regard to volume status.

248. Answer: B

Answer: Na 115, K 5.2, Cl 82, CO$_2$ 21, BUN 12, Cr 1.0, Glu 98, pH 7.34, Urine Na 43.
This represents hyponatremia, with mild hyperkalemia, no pre-renal azotemia, and urinary sodium losses. This is most consistent with Addison disease, in which case mineralocorticoid deficiency results in potassium retention.

Board Testing Point: Recognize the electrolyte and laboratory abnormalities associated with Addison disease.

249. Answer: C

Answer: Na 115, K 3.2, Cl 72, CO$_2$ 31, BUN 45, Cr 1.0, Glu 101, pH 7.47, Urine Na 43.
There is a metabolic alkalosis, pre-renal azotemia, and urine sodium losses. The urine sodium is high because bicarbonate in the urine acts as a non-resorbable anion in the tubule and takes sodium with it. In metabolic alkalosis, therefore, it is important to measure urinary chloride which would be low.

Board Testing Point: Recognize the electrolyte and laboratory abnormalities associated with acute vomiting.

250. Answer: E

Answer: Na 115, K 3.2, Cl 82, CO$_2$ 21, BUN 45, Cr 1.6, Glu 89, pH 7.34, Urine Na 11.
This patient has a hypokalemic metabolic acidosis and pre-renal azotemia, but is retaining sodium. This is most consistent with volume depletion secondary to diarrhea, where losses contain primarily bicarbonate. These patients may also have a non-anion gap metabolic acidosis, and if there is any question as to whether the patient has an RTA or diarrhea, one could measure the urinary anion gap, which will be positive in patients with GI bicarbonate losses, since they are able to generate NH4.

Board Testing Point: Recognize the electrolyte and laboratory abnormalities associated with prolonged diarrhea.

251. Answer: E

Answer: Na 115, K 3.2, Cl 72, CO$_2$ 24, BUN 12 Cr 1.0, Glu 89, pH 7.40, Urine Na 43.
Patients with hyponatremia may also be euvolemic, as in SIADH. The differential diagnosis includes psychogenic polydipsia, glucocorticoid deficiency, and hypothyroidism. In the patient with SIADH, there should not be evidence of acid-base disturbance or pre-renal azotemia.

Board Testing Point: Recognize the electrolyte and laboratory abnormalities associated with SIADH.

252. Answer: A

Answer: BP 162/98, Na 132, K 3.2, CO_2 34, Cl 80, Scr 1.1, pH 7.44, PCO_2 44, HCO_3 33, UCl 32, Urine pH 7.6.
These findings represent a hypertensive patient with a hypokalemic metabolic alkalosis. Metabolic alkalosis can be classified as low or high urine chloride. In this case, the urine chloride is high; therefore, the patient is likely to have either steroid excess, including hyperaldosteronism or Bartter syndrome. Since this patient is hypertensive, the diagnosis is most likely primary hyperaldosteronism, and he is likely to improve with spironolactone.

Board Testing Point: Recognize the clinical and laboratory abnormalities associated with primary hyperaldosteronism.

253. Answer: B

Answer: BP 120/80, Na 132, K 3.2, CO_2 34, Cl 80, Scr 1.1, pH 7.44, PCO_2 44, HCO_3 33, UCl 32, Urine pH 7.6.
Patients with Bartter syndrome have a metabolic alkalosis with a high urine chloride. They also have normal blood pressure and should be treated with a prostaglandin inhibitor, indomethacin.

Board Testing Point: Recognize the clinical and laboratory abnormalities associated with Bartter syndrome.

254. Answer: C

Answer: BP 120/80, Na 132, K 3.2, CO_2 34, Cl 80, Scr 1.1, pH 7.44, PCO_2 44, HCO_3 33, UCl 8, Urine pH 7.6.
This patient has a hypokalemic, metabolic alkalosis, and is normotensive. However, the urine chloride is low, suggesting volume depletion. Causes for this include vomiting, nasogastric suction, or diuretics.

Board Testing Point: Recognize the clinical and laboratory abnormalities associated with prolonged nasogastric tube use.

255. Answer: D

Answer: BP 120/80, Na 132, K 3.2, CO_2 16, Cl 104, Scr 1.1, pH 7.34, PCO_2 35, HCO_3 18, UCl 32, Urine pH 7.6.
In RTA type I, you have a patient with a non-anion gap, hypokalemic metabolic acidosis. The most common disorders that do this are either renal tubular acidosis or diarrhea. While the history will usually establish the diagnosis, one could also use the urine anion gap if the urinary Na, K, and Cl are known. In patients with diarrhea, the kidney acidifies the urine appropriately and generates NH4; therefore the urine Cl increases and the urine AG becomes positive. In this case, the urine pH is high, consistent with Type I RTA, a disorder known to be associated with hypercalciuria and nephrolithiasis.

Board Testing Point: Recognize the clinical and laboratory abnormalities associated with Type I RTA.

256. Answer: E

Answer: BP 120/80, Na 132, K 3.2, CO_2 16, Cl 104, Scr 1.1, pH 7.34, PCO_2 35, HCO_3 18, UCl 32, Urine pH 5.4.
Here you have a patient with presumed chronic diarrhea and you expect to find a non-anion gap, hypokalemic metabolic acidosis. The most common disorders that do this are either renal tubular acidosis or diarrhea. While the history will usually establish the diagnosis, one could also use the urine anion gap if the urinary Na, K, and Cl are known. In patients with diarrhea, the kidney acidifies the urine appropriately and generates NH_4; therefore the urine Cl increases and the urine AG becomes positive. The pH is helpful in differentiating diarrhea from RTA type I because in RTA Type I the pH cannot be below 5.5.

Board Testing Point: Recognize the clinical and laboratory abnormalities associated with prolonged diarrhea and laxative abuse.

257. Answer: E

Answer: BP 120/80, Na 132, K 4.6, CO_2 16, Cl 94, Scr 1.1, pH 7.38, PCO_2 30, HCO_3 18, UCl 32, Urine pH 5.4.
This patient has an anion gap metabolic acidosis. If one applies the "Winter formula," the pCO_2 should be 35 (1.5 $\times HCO_3$ + 8). This patient has a pCO_2 of 30; therefore, the patient is hyperventilating and has a superimposed respiratory alkalosis. Disorders that can cause this mixed acid-base disorder include sepsis and salicylate intoxication.

Board Testing Point: Recognize the clinical and laboratory abnormalities associated with aspirin toxicity.

258. Answer: B

Answer: BP 120/80, Na 132, K 5.2, CO_2 16, Cl 104, Scr 2.1, pH 7.34, PCO_2 35, HCO_3 18, UCl 32, Urine pH 5.4.
This represents a scenario of non-anion gap hyperkalemic metabolic acidosis with abnormal renal function. Similar to a patient with Type I RTA, this patient also has an RTA, but is distinguished by the hyperkalemia and the low urine pH. This is consistent with a Type IV RTA, most commonly found in diabetics with mild renal disease. Treatment can include a low potassium diet, fludrocortisone, oral bicarbonate therapy and/or diuretics.

Board Testing Point: Recognize the clinical and laboratory abnormalities associated with Type IV RTA.

259. Answer: C

Answer: Hydrochlorothiazide, a total of 50 mg a day.
Several medications and chemicals influence uric acid excretion. Thiazide diuretics inhibit renal excretion of uric acid, so serum levels of uric acid rise. High-dose aspirin, > 2000 mg a day, increases uric acid excretion and lowers the serum levels of uric acid. Low-dose aspirin, even 81 mg a day, inhibits the excretion, and hence raises the serum levels of uric acid. Methotrexate, ibuprofen, and mycophenolate do not have any effect on serum uric acid levels.

Board Testing Point: Diuretics, especially the thiazides, alcohol, low-dose aspirin, and cyclosporine inhibit renal excretion of uric acid and should be avoided in patients with significant hyperuricemia whenever possible.

260. Answer: A

Answer: Glomerulonephritis.
Red blood cell casts are formed when bleeding occurs in the nephron and casts are formed in the collecting tubules. Bleeding from the ureters, bladder and urethra does not form these casts. Of the options noted, glomerulonephritis is the only process directly related to bleeding within the nephron.

Board Testing Point: Identify the significance of red blood cell casts.

ENDOCRINOLOGY

261. Answer: D

Answer: ACTH-producing tumor.
The patient's clinical findings are consistent with Cushing disease. She has moon facies, buffalo hump, central obesity, and striae. She also demonstrates hyperpigmentation. An ACTH-producing tumor displays both increased levels of ACTH, which drives hyperpigmentation and stimulates increased levels of cortisol production. Primary adrenal failure stimulates increased production of ACTH, which can lead to hyperpigmentation. These patients, however, have decreased cortisol levels. Adrenal hyperplasia produces increased levels of cortisol, but ACTH levels are suppressed and hyperpigmentation is not a component of this process. Secondary adrenal failure arises from decreased ACTH leading to diminished cortisol production, and would lack both hypercortisolism as well as hyperpigmentation.

Board Testing Point: Diagnose Cushing disease based on clinical findings and identify the most likely etiology.

262. Answer: B

Answer: Prescribe thyroid supplementation to suppress TSH and maintain free T$_4$ levels in the high-normal range.
Most thyroid cancers retain responsiveness to TSH stimulation, and thyroid supplements are an important component of thyroid cancer treatment. The goal is to suppress TSH levels, and thereby TSH stimulation of potential residual tumor cells as low as possible without inducing the side effects associated with hyperthyroidism. These effects include cardiac, bone, and psychological manifestations. Deliberate induction of hyperthyroidism is not appropriate, and acceptance of hypothyroidism with increased TSH would be detrimental to the patient. The most appropriate intervention is thyroid supplements to suppress TSH and maintain free T4 levels in the high-normal range as tolerated.

Board Testing Point: Synthesize the reasoning behind TSH suppression in the treatment of thyroid cancers.

263. Answer: A

Answer: Adrenal tumor.
Hypertension that presents with hypokalemia and metabolic alkalosis is suggestive of a mineralocorticoid excess, resulting in potassium wasting. Distinguishing the etiology of the hypokalemia and hypertension can be aided by measurement of plasma aldosterone levels and plasma renin activity. Aldosterone levels are normally regulated primarily by the renin-angiotensin system and, to a lesser extent, by ACTH stimulation and serum potassium levels. Patients with primary hyperaldosteronism have increased plasma aldosterone levels that result in suppression of plasma renin activity, as noted in this scenario. Adrenal hyperplasia and adrenal tumors are the most frequent causes of this condition.

Bartter syndrome is caused by a defect leading to renal salt wasting, which leads to hypovolemia and stimulating both increased renin production and subsequent increases in aldosterone levels. These patients show hypokalemia but do not tend to have hypertension. Liddle syndrome is an autosomal dominant defect in renal sodium channels that allow retention of sodium, leading to potassium wasting and hypertension. The increased volume related to sodium retention suppresses both renin and aldosterone levels. In patients with secondary aldosterone, the plasma renin is significantly increased, resulting in an increase in aldosterone. Conditions such as renal artery stenosis, volume contraction from diuretics, and renin-producing tumors are associated with secondary hyperaldosteronism.

Board Testing Point: Interpret laboratory tests and identify an adrenal tumor as a cause of secondary hypertension.

---

264. Answer: A

Answer: Acetaminophen.
Hyperthermia in hyperthyroidism is a common feature and contributes to the hypermetabolic status. Reducing the temperature elevation reduces the metabolic demands and can provide symptomatic improvement for the patient. Both aspirin and non-steroidal antiinflammatory medications increase the release of thyroid from bonding globulins and enhance active thyroid levels. Acetaminophen does not have this effect and is the best initial antipyretic. Dantrolene is useful in neuroleptic malignant syndrome, but it is not indicated in this scenario.

Board Testing Point: Prescribe the appropriate antipyretic in the setting of a hyperthyroid febrile state.

---

265. Answer: C

Answer: Lab error.
Glucose is the basic energy source for the brain, and diminished supply results in decreased neuronal performance. Some disease states can blunt a person's sensitivity to peripheral manifestations of hypoglycemia, but mental function is compromised in all patients with prolonged restriction of glucose supply.

A completely asymptomatic person is unlikely to have a significant hypoglycemic state. An insulinoma, surreptitious insulin usage, anorexia, and adrenal insufficiency are all conditions that may manifest with hypoglycemia, but these patients would demonstrate cognitive impairment if the glucose was 35 mg/dL. Metabolic processes of the cellular components of blood can continue to consume glucose after a blood specimen has been collected. High cell counts (polycythemia, leukocytosis, etc.), delay in processing the specimen, or failure to spin the specimen and separate the cellular component from the serum can result in falsely depressed glucose levels.

Board Review Point: Identify a laboratory error as an etiology of reported hypoglycemia.

---

266. Answer: D

Answer: Hypomagnesemia.
Hypomagnesemia is common in patients with alcoholism (up to 30% of hospitalized alcoholic patients) and interferes with parathyroid function (suppresses PTH secretion and causes resistance at the receptor level to the actions of PTH). Severe hypomagnesemia is usually noted by signs and symptoms of hypocalcemia (Chvostek sign, Trousseau sign), but may also cause seizures, malabsorption, bone disease, and cardiac arrhythmias. Alcoholism interferes with tubular absorption/reabsorption of magnesium. In addition, alcoholic patients have diets poor in magnesium and may have steatorrhea and/or pancreatitis, which also may lead to severe hypomagnesemia. The picture is of a telangiectasia, common in alcoholic patients. Hypomagnesemia is common while the other choices are rare.

Board Testing Point: Interpret the clinical findings of hypocalcemia and attribute them to hypomagnesemia based on a clinical history.

267. Answer: B

Answer: Gynecomastia.
Exogenous androgens suppress normal gonadotropin release and decrease testicular function, including sperm counts. Long-term use can also lead to reduction in testicular size. Androgens are associated with erythropoietic stimulation, and elevated red blood cell counts are typically found in androgen abuse. Normal physiological levels of androgens are sufficient for full virilization effects in males, and supplemental hormones do not cause increased masculinization. The increased levels also do not reduce virilization or directly affect hair distribution, but do increase acne formation, especially on the chest and back (as shown in the picture). Increased testosterone levels are converted to estradiol, which can lead to gynecomastia. This effect is limited to androgens, like testosterone, that can be metabolized to estradiol. Other androgens that do not convert to estradiol therefore will not lead to this effect.

Board Testing Point: Know the findings of exogenous testosterone abuse and, on the Board exam, be suspicious for abuse in an adolescent male with aggressive, abnormal behavior.

268. Answer: E

Answer: Low TSH, elevated free T4, low uptake on thyroid scan.
Thyroiditis may be relatively asymptomatic, but often presents as transient hyperthyroidism. Thyroid follicles are destroyed, releasing thyroid hormone and causing hyperthyroid signs and symptoms; but uptake scanning shows diminished uptake since the affected thyroid follicles are nonfunctional. Free T4 levels are elevated (released from the thyroid gland); TSH is suppressed by the elevated T4.

Board Testing Point: Predict derangements of thyroid function tests and abnormalities of the thyroid scan in a setting of transient hyperthyroidism.

269. Answer: B

Answer: Potassium.
Hypokalemia is strongly correlated with low serum magnesium levels. The next best answer would be calcium, because low magnesium levels may affect PTH release and could lower calcium levels. This correlation is not as strong as the reduction in potassium levels seen with hypomagnesemia. Sodium, potassium, and creatinine are not affected by low magnesium levels.

Board Testing Point: Synthesize the most common electrolyte abnormalities associated with derangements in magnesium.

270. Answer: D

Answer: Medullary thyroid cancer.
The disease processes noted in this patient's kinship include medullary thyroid cancer, pheochromocytoma, and hyperparathyroidism. The picture is showing a calcium oxalate crystal consistent with calcium oxalate stone formation in a patient with hyperparathyroidism. This group of abnormalities is consistent with Multiple Endocrine Neoplasia (MEN) 2A. Individuals with this syndrome have a predilection for medullary thyroid cancer, and the course in these patients is usually more aggressive then in non-MEN patients. Pancreatic abnormalities (insulinoma, gastrinoma) and pituitary lesions (prolactinoma) are more common in MEN 1. MEN

2B manifests neuromas, medullary thyroid cancer, and pheochromocytoma, but parathyroid disease is not part of this subgroup.

Board Testing Point: Recall the clinical conditions featured in MEN 2B and predict their presence based on interpretation of laboratory data.

271. Answer: D

Answer: Stop glipizide and reduce the dose of rosiglitazone.
It is assumed that every diabetic will need insulin eventually. This does not mean that your patients get started on insulin because they have "failed." On the contrary, being controlled for a period of time with oral drugs alone is an accomplishment. However, diabetes is a relentless disease and beta-cell failure worsens over time. The triple combination of a sulfonylurea, metformin, and a thiazolidinedione is common. But the need for insulin is even more common.

Nocturnal NPH insulin is often used in combination with insulin secretagogues with great success, but there is little need for an insulin secretagogue after starting bolus insulin. Insulin is approved in combination with the thiazolidinediones, but not at the maximum dose of either rosiglitazone or pioglitazone because of an increased risk for heart failure. This patient's rosiglitazone can be continued after adding insulin, but the dose needs to be decreased. Metformin is also approved in combination with insulin. Although it doesn't really lead to weight loss, it can significantly ameliorate the expected weight gain after adding insulin. In addition, the insulin sensitizers (metformin and thiazolidinediones) will decrease the dose of insulin needed by the patient, because they reduce insulin resistance. The best choice among the listed options is to discontinue glipizide, continue metformin at its current dose, and continue rosiglitazone but at a reduced dose. Once his glycemic control has improved, the rosiglitazone may be discontinued to make his treatment regimen less complicated.

Board Testing Point: Assemble a regimen for treating hyperglycemia in a patient with complicated diabetes.

272. Answer: E

Answer: E. Stop the thiazolidinedione, begin monitoring glucose very carefully, start basal and bolus insulin with NPH and regular insulin, and refer her to an obstetrician with experience in high-risk pregnancies.
The only drugs approved for the treatment of diabetes during pregnancy are human insulins. Metformin and thiazolidinediones are absolutely contraindicated. The sulfonylureas appear to be safe but have not yet been approved in pregnancy. The insulin analogues are also expected to be approved one day but are not yet available for pregnant patients. The standard treatment of diabetes during pregnancy is very careful monitoring of glucose levels, very consistent meals, and human NPH and regular insulin. Diabetics are prone to have complications during pregnancy and must be followed by an experienced obstetrician.

Board Testing Point: Prescribe an appropriate regimen to manage diabetes in a pregnancy.

273. Answer: A

Answer: Excess iodine.
Although excess iodine can lead to either hypothyroidism or hyperthyroidism, it can also cause a euthyroid goiter. Iodine is present in iodized salt, and typical intake results in normal iodine concentrations. Excess iodine typically results when patients inadvertently increase their intake by doubling up on iodine-specific supplements and multivitamins. Excess TSH will stimulate the thyroid gland and cause a hyperthyroid goiter. Excess TRH

will lead to the same outcome, because it will stimulate excess secretion of TSH. Excessive exogenous T3 and a struma ovarii would be expected to result in hyperthyroidism without a goiter.

Board Testing Point: Interpret thyroid function tests and identify iodine excess as an etiology of a euthyroid goiter.

274. Answer: A

Answer: TC 321, LDL 265, HDL 34, TG 110.
Individuals with heterozygous familial hypercholesterolemia have a 50% reduction in LDL receptor activity. Their LDL cholesterol levels are roughly doubled and usually fall within the range of 190-350 mg/dL. On the exam, one would expect the LDL to exceed 250 mg/dL.

Board Testing Point: Predict the lipid profile for a patient with heterozygous familial hypercholesterolemia.

275. Answer: B

Answer: Refer him to nuclear medicine for radioablation.
A hot nodule does not need to be biopsied, because the risk of it containing cancer is extraordinarily low. Exogenous thyroxine will not suppress the nodule and will only make him more hyperthyroid. PTU could be used to treat his hyperthyroidism, but it is not a long-term solution. The best course of action is to refer him for ablation.

Board Testing Point: Construct a management plan for a hot thyroid nodule.

276. Answer: E

Answer: All of the choices are possible.
It is estimated that 10% of amiodarone is bioavailable iodine. This far exceeds our daily iodine needs. Amiodarone can affect thyroid function by providing a large excess of iodine. This iodine load can either cause hypothyroidism or hyperthyroidism. Amiodarone can also cause a thyroiditis, and this thyroiditis can be accompanied by either hypothyroidism or hyperthyroidism.

Board Testing Point: Summarize the types of thyroid disease associated with amiodarone use.

277. Answer: E

Answer: Both primary hyperaldosteronism and Cushing syndrome.
All four disorders may cause hypertension with a hypokalemic metabolic alkalosis. The underlying etiology is excess aldosterone. Plasma renin activity levels are low in primary hyperaldosteronism and Cushing syndrome while high in renal artery stenosis and cases of reninoma.

Board Testing Point: Recognize the findings of hypertension with a hypokalemic metabolic alkalosis, and then be able to differentiate the etiology based on the renin level.

278. Answer: A

Answer: Cushing disease.
All of these can cause hypertension except Cushing disease. This refers to a pituitary tumor secreting ACTH. Although both adrenal glands become enlarged, they do not develop adenomas. An adrenal tumor secreting cortisol is an example of Cushing syndrome.

Board Testing Point: Recognize that Cushing disease does not cause hypertension.

279. Answer: C

Answer: Hungry bone syndrome.
Hyperparathyroidism is often present for an extended period of time because of a lack of early symptoms. Patients can experience significant demineralization of their bones. After removal of the parathyroid adenoma, the PTH levels initially drop, and the bones avidly take up calcium and phosphate. If this process is particularly avid, the serum levels of calcium and phosphate can decrease significantly. The normal parathyroid glands are still intact, and they will begin to secrete PTH in an attempt to raise the calcium level. The patient needs to be given calcium supplementation. Eventually, the bones will have replaced much of the lost calcium, and serum calcium levels will return to normal, along with PTH and phosphate. At this point, the calcium supplements can be stopped. The other choices do not fit the laboratory findings listed.

Board Testing Point: Identify the hungry bone syndrome based on clinical history and laboratory data.

280. Answer: A

Answer: 11ß-hydroxysteroid dehydrogenase type 2.
Natural licorice contains glycyrrhetinic acid, which leads to inhibition of 11ß-hydroxysteroid dehydrogenase type 2. This enzyme converts cortisol into cortisone within the kidney. Cortisol activates the mineralocorticoid receptor, but cortisone does not. By blocking this enzyme, cortisol is not converted into cortisone within the kidney, and the cortisol leads to excess activation of the mineralocorticoid receptor. The other enzymes listed are not associated with licorice ingestion.

Board Testing Point: Associate licorice with hypertension (a FAVORITE board question).

281. Answer: A

Answer: 21α-hydroxylase.
Most causes of late-onset congenital adrenal hyperplasia are very rare, but 21α-hydroxylase is relatively common. This enzymatic deficiency is seen in about 1 per 12,000, and 1-2 % are carriers.

Board Testing Point: Identify 21α-hydroxylase as the most common cause of last-onset congenital adrenal hyperplasia.

282. Answer: C

Answer: A pituitary tumor secreting TSH.
The thyroid-stimulating immunoglobulins of Grave disease would continue to stimulate any remaining thyroid tissue, including a struma ovarii or thyroid tissue not resected by the surgeon. Excess thyroid hormone T4 or T3 would also maintain hyperthyroidism. If the thyroid gland is removed, then any TSH secreted by a pituitary tumor would not cause hyperthyroidism.

Board Testing Point: Recognize that, with thyroidectomy, a pituitary tumor that secretes TSH would not have its target organ (the thyroid gland is now removed), and thyroid levels should not be elevated.

283. Answer: A

Answer: Sweating.
Nonselective beta-blockers can block many of the signs and symptoms of hypoglycemia except for those mediated by the cholinergic system. Sweating is stimulated by cholinergic nerves and should not be blocked by nonselective beta-blockers. The other manifestations of hypoglycemia are often blocked by these drugs.

Board Testing Point: Recognize the interaction between nonselective beta-blockers and the signs and symptoms of hypoglycemia.

284. Answer: E

Answer: Lower risk of developing retinopathy.
Tight control of insulin-treated type 2 diabetes clearly reduces the risk of developing the microvascular complications of diabetes, which are nephropathy, neuropathy, and retinopathy. Tight control also reduces serum levels of triglycerides. However, we do not yet have trials that clearly demonstrate a reduction in the risk of developing cardiovascular disease with tight glycemic control. The evidence is tantalizing but not statistically significant at the p < 0.05 level. The UKPDS trial almost found significance, but the *P* value was 0.052, which is greater than 0.05; therefore considered nonsignificant. We all await further trials addressing this issue.

Board Testing Point: Recognize that tight control of insulin-treated type 2 DM results in reduced risk of nephropathy, neuropathy, and retinopathy.

285. Answer: B

Answer: Check liver function tests within 8-12 weeks.
When encountering an elevated LDL cholesterol level, it is important to ask the patient about diet compliance. If the statin dose is increased, the liver function tests should be checked in 8-12 weeks. Any patient taking a statin needs to be reminded of the possible side effects, including muscle aches. Hypothyroidism can cause an elevated level of LDL cholesterol, but is not usually tested in an asymptomatic individual with no clinical signs or history of thyroid disease. Checking a CPK level is not routine in an asymptomatic patient but is clearly indicated if muscle aches develop.

Board Testing Point: Arrange appropriate laboratory testing when increasing a statin medication because of possible side effects.

286. Answer: E

Answer: Ovarian cysts.
The diagnosis of PCOS centers on the presence of hyperandrogenism and irregular menses. LH is usually increased, while FSH is usually normal, and this results in an elevated LH/FSH ratio. In PCOS, the typical LH/FSH ratio is greater than 3, but both hormones levels may be normal, so a ratio of less than 3 does not exclude the diagnosis. Glucose intolerance is also generally seen in this disorder. The ultrasound would characteristically show > 8 cysts in each ovary (some say greater than 12 follicles ranging in size 2-9 mm).

Board Testing Point: Recognize the diagnostic findings for polycystic ovary disease.

287. Answer: B

Answer: Type 1 diabetes mellitus.
Type 2 diabetes is not characterized by autoimmune destruction of the beta cells. Type 1 diabetes is most often caused by autoimmune destruction of these insulin-secreting cells. Primary adrenal insufficiency and vitiligo are also autoimmune in nature, but are not characterized by destruction of the beta cells.

Board Testing Point: Recognize that type 1 diabetes mellitus is most often due to autoimmune destruction of beta cells.

288. Answer: E

Answer: Worsened retinopathy, even with tight glucose control.
Pre-pregnancy counseling is very important for any diabetic woman contemplating pregnancy. Sulfonylureas are not approved for pregnant women, and the other oral drugs are absolutely contraindicated in pregnancy. Her only option is insulin, and this is currently limited to regular and NPH human insulin. Tight control is vital for fetal development. Very consistent meals and frequent glucose checking will facilitate control. It is also important to achieve tight glucose control before conception. If she can maintain tight control, the risk for the other fetal complications listed, including macrosomia, is greatly reduced. Unfortunately, maternal retinopathy often worsens even with this tight control.

Board Testing Point: Identify retinopathy as a condition that can worsen during pregnancy in a diabetic.

289. Answer: E

Answer: Ethanol intoxication.
Primary adrenal insufficiency, pheochromocytoma, and insulin overdose may all cause hypoglycemia. Ethanol can cause hypoglycemia because it blocks hepatic gluconeogenesis, and hypoglycemia occurs after glycogen stores are exhausted. This is worsened by the person's inability to recognize hypoglycemia and to take corrective actions, usually because of decreased consciousness. Given this patient's history and negative review of systems, this is the most likely diagnosis. Hypoglycemia is common with beta-cell tumors, such as insulinomas, but is not associated with alpha-cell tumors such as glucagonomas.

Board Testing Point: Differentiate the etiologies of hypoglycemia.

290. Answer: A

Answer: Counsel the patient that getting pregnant is more difficult if she is not euthyroid, because she is more likely to have irregular menses.
Once pregnant, she will need a larger dose of thyroxine, and this can be reduced to the pre-pregnancy dose after delivery. High estrogen levels in pregnancy do stimulate the liver to produce many different proteins, including TBG, but thyroxine doses must be adjusted carefully based on laboratory monitoring, as opposed to simply doubling the pre-pregnancy dose. Correction of maternal hypothyroidism can benefit the child's IQ, and strict adherence to thyroxine supplementation during pregnancy should be encouraged.

Board Testing Point: Forecast the changes that occur in thyroid hormone levels during pregnancy.

291. Answer: A

Answer: Hypercalcemia.
Hypercalcemia is most commonly caused by hyperparathyroidism or malignancy (usually breast or lung cancer or multiple myeloma), but can also be caused by sarcoidosis and other granulomatous diseases.

When caused by hyperparathyroidism, the hypercalcemia is usually mild; this is also known as primary hyperparathyroidism. This occurs more often in women, and its incidence increases with age. The increase in calcium is due to the hypersecretion of parathyroid hormone (PTH), which causes an increase in the absorption of calcium in the intestine, as well as decreased excretion of calcium at the renal tubule. The osteoclasts in the bones are not involved in this process.

When caused by cancer, the hypercalcemia is usually more severe. It is due to increased osteoclastic activity within the bone (non-PTH mediated). This affects men and women equally, and increases in incidence with increasing age (as does the occurrence of these tumors).

Symptoms of hypercalcemia include nausea, vomiting, abdominal pain, altered mentation, and lethargy. Some patients report muscle and joint pains. Physical findings include hyperreflexia and tongue fasciculations. Laboratory testing shows elevated calcium. An ECG shows a prolonged QT, shortened PR, and may show heart block. When calcium levels are very high, the QRS complex may widen.

The treatment is to rapidly correct the hypercalcemia. The prognosis depends on the underlying cause. If caused by a malignancy, the prognosis is usually poor.

Hyperkalemia can also cause a shortened QT on ECG and a widened QRS, but also causes hyporeflexia. Hypocalcemia, hypokalemia, and carbon monoxide poisoning do not produce these ECG changes.

Board Testing Point: Recognize the clinical findings of hypercalcemia and interpret an electrocardiogram showing a widened QRS complex and a prolonged QT interval.

292. Answer: E

Answer: All of the choices are correct.
The most common causes of increased serum calcium are primary hyperparathyroidism (PTH level) and cancer (skeletal survey). Both increase in incidence with age; therefore, both are possible here. In addition, sarcoid (CXR) and pancreatitis (amylase and lipase) can cause an elevation in serum calcium, and should be evaluated. In other words, all of these possibilities need to be investigated.

293. Answer: C

Answer: Ketoacidosis.

Ketoacidosis occurs more often in juvenile diabetes, and is due to insulin deficiency. The body cannot utilize serum glucose, and breaks down fat as a fuel source, generating ketones. These can create a "fruity" smell to the breath as they are excreted through the oral mucosa. Physical symptoms may include polyuria and polydipsia, abdominal pain, nausea, and vomiting. Rapid, deep breathing may also occur.

Nonketotic/hyperosmolar states may present with similar symptoms, but occur much more often in adult-onset diabetes (our patient is an adolescent), in a person who either forgets to take their insulin, eats sugary meals, or neglects to drink an appropriate amount of liquid. Hypoglycemia causes tremulousness, sweating, and hunger in association with lethargy.

The treatment of ketoacidosis and hyperosmolar states are fluids, insulin, and repletion of electrolytes (sodium and potassium). Hypoglycemia is treated with glucose or glucagons, a hormone that causes the release of glucose from the body's glucose stores. Without further symptoms or explanation, pancreatitis and hypercalcemia would be rare in a young woman.

Board Testing Point: Diagnose ketoacidosis based on a history and clinical examination.

294. Answer: B

Answer: Secondary hypothyroidism.

This patient presents with classic symptoms of hypothyroidism. Clinically, she shows no apparent goiter. Measurement of decreased free T_4 is consistent with hypothyroidism. In primary hypothyroidism (failure of the thyroid gland), the TSH elevates to stimulate the gland to "produce more, more, more!" In this scenario however, the TSH is low. Therefore, this is not a case of primary hypothyroidism. A low T4 and low TSH occurs in cases of secondary hypothyroidism associated with pituitary gland failure. Tertiary hypothyroidism is associated with diminished secretion of thyroid releasing hormone (TRH) from the hypothalamus resulting in lowered TSH levels. But, in this case, we do not give you TRH levels. So, you have to ascertain if the pituitary is functioning by interpreting the FSH level. A patient in menopause should display significantly elevated FSH levels, so the low FSH level is suggestive of diminished pituitary function. Therefore, this case is most consistent with secondary hypothyroidism. Anti-thyroid antibodies are often, but not always, associated with a goiter. The effects of the antibodies may cause both hypo- and hyper-thyroid conditions, but the TSH feedback loop remains intact.

Board Testing Point: Interpret testing of the pituitary gland to identify secondary hypothyroidism.

295. Answer: D

Answer: MRI of the head with contrast.

Carefully review the case, making a list of all of the problems:
1. median nerve entrapment, left hand
2. newly diagnosed diabetes
3. headaches with decreased visual acuity and a visual field defect
4. coarsening of features
5. decreased libido
6. recent diagnosis of hypertension

This collection of problems is consistent with a pituitary tumor causing acromegaly. It would be inappropriate to simply diagnose the diabetes, institute treatment, attribute the carpal tunnel syndrome to diabetes only and ignore the visual field defect and decreased libido. The carpal tunnel can be diagnosed by history and physical exam, and an EMG study is unnecessary. Any patient with weight gain and a new diagnosis of diabetes should be considered a candidate for Cushing disease or syndrome. However, in this case, the other findings distinctly point to the pituitary as a site for pathology, and the physical exam is more consistent with acromegaly than cortisol excess. Thyroid disease is much less likely than acromegaly.

Acromegaly is most commonly caused by a tumor in the anterior pituitary that secretes growth hormone. The tumor-mass effect is responsible for the local symptoms of headache, reduced visual acuity, and visual field defects. Symptoms of acromegaly are very subtle, and patients usually are not diagnosed until a median of 12 years after the symptoms start! The most dramatic manifestations occur in the soft tissues with macrognathia and enlargement of the hands and feet. Asking this patient whether his shoe and shirt sizes have increased in the past few years is helpful. Foreheads enlarge and the teeth often spread out. Arthralgias and back pain are common due to the enlargement of synovium and cartilage. This patient's hypertension and displaced PMI is likely related to the acromegaly since both are associated (left ventricular hypertrophy is common). Hypogonadism due to mass effect is also common, and male patients typically have decreased libido, often with reduced erections, and most women have disruption of menses. Evaluation for acromegaly should proceed in patients with signs and symptoms and should include 1) assessment for growth hormone excess (using serum GH and IGF-I concentrations) and 2) radiologic search for a pituitary adenoma.

Board Testing Point: Diagnose acromegaly based on complicated history, physical findings and labs and order the appropriate study for evaluation of the anterior pituitary.

296. Answer: C

Answer: Levothyroxine 50 mcg daily.
This is a classic case of hypothyroidism in an elderly patient with co-morbid heart disease. The diagnosis can be clearly made by evaluating the elevated TSH level in the setting of a low free T4 level. Replacing thyroid hormone in such a patient is tricky because of the increase in myocardial oxygen demand precipitated by thyroid hormone. Elderly patients on rapid replacement are more likely to experience arrhythmias, angina, and myocardial infarction. Therefore, 50 mcg of levothyroxine daily is the recommended starting dose (regardless of kg body weight) for patients aged > 50 years and in patients with documented CAD. For other patients, the recommended starting dose is 1.6 mcg/kg body weight per day, using lean body mass. Liothyronine is the generic name for a T3 replacement product; T3 replacement is not recommended because of the instability of the preparation and its short half-life.

Board Testing Point: Prescribe the appropriate dose of thyroid hormone replacement in an elderly patient with coronary artery disease.

297. Answer: B

Answer: Pituitary apoplexy.
This is a case of a prolactinoma, as evidenced by oligomenorrhea, visual field defects, and galactorrhea. In patients with pituitary tumors, a headache that is retroorbital, severe, and acute is concerning for pituitary apoplexy, a condition that can occur when the tumor outgrows its blood supply or infarcts. The infarction leads to subsequent hemorrhage into the gland with swelling, causing headache and neurologic impairment. The neurologic symptoms range from none to mental status disturbances. Most patients will present with headache, and 69% will have associated vomiting. The prolactinoma itself is not causing the sudden onset headache, but it is responsible for the long-term visual field defects. Subarachnoid hemorrhage and migraine are possibilities but

would not be associated with the hypogonadism consistent with a preexisting pituitary adenoma. In patients with headache, the review of systems is very important in ascertaining whether a mass lesion is present. Cerebrovascular accident would be very rare in a 32-year-old woman.

Board Testing Point: Interpret a history and physical exam to diagnose a pituitary adenoma; identify apoplexy as the etiology of an acute, severe headache in a patient with symptoms of an adenoma.

---

298. Answer: A

Answer: Observation with repeat of thyroid functions after this acute illness.
This is a case of sick-euthyroid syndrome. In most patients with a severe acute illness (often requiring the ICU), thyroid function studies are measured as abnormal, although no clinical disease exists. TSH, total T3, and T4 levels can all be low, but most patients do not have pituitary disease. Therefore, it is important to measure thyroid functions only in sick patients with significant evidence of thyroid dysfunction (e.g., atrial fibrillation = hyperthyroidism or myxedema = hypothyroidism). Ancillary testing can differentiate whether this patient has central hypothyroidism due to pituitary dysfunction, but further tests are unnecessary in settings where true symptoms of hypothyroidism are absent. The patient described has a slow heart rate and some weight gain, but both symptoms can be explained by his age and his recent involvement in athletic activity. He has no physical examination findings consistent with thyroid disease.

Heparin injections can affect thyroid function studies by decreasing the binding of T4 to thyroid binding globulin (TBG). Other medications also affect the thyroid function tests without actually affecting thyroid function, including glucocorticoids, methadone/heroin, certain NSAIDS, dopamine, dobutamine, amiodarone and a number of others. However, the state of "sick euthyroid" is not dangerous and does not require discontinuation of necessary medications in order to normalize laboratory tests.

Most patients with low but detectable TSH have normal thyroid function studies when the tests are repeated after resolution of the acute illness.

Board testing point: Interpret thyroid functions and diagnose sick-euthyroid syndrome.

HEMATOLOGY

299. Answer: C

Answer: 6 six months of oral warfarin plus B vitamins (folate, B-6, B-12).
Hyperhomocysteinemia may reflect B complex vitamin deficiency (folate, B-6, B-12) and is associated with both arterial (premature CAD) and venous thrombosis. B vitamin supplementation should be initiated in patients with hyperhomocysteinemia, especially in the setting of thromboembolic disease. The current recommendation for duration of anticoagulation following a first idiopathic thromboembolic event is six months (three months if there was a time-limited, reversible risk factor, e.g., surgery). Age-appropriate cancer screening should be done after a first thrombosis. In patients with recurrent thrombosis, the chance of underlying malignancy is increased, so a more intensified search for underlying malignancy might be warranted. IVC filters are used in patients who fail anticoagulation or have a contraindication to anticoagulation.

Board Testing Point: Institute treatment for hyperhomocysteinemia-associated thrombosis.

300. Answer: B

Answer: von Willebrand disease.
Of the options listed, only von Willebrand disease will give you a normal PT, elevated PTT, normal CBC, elevated bleeding time, and abnormal RIPA. Remember that vitamin K deficiency and Factor VII deficiency will give you an abnormal PT. Bernard-Soulier syndrome is the giant platelet syndrome. Factor XIII deficiency has a normal PT and PTT.

Board Testing Point: Diagnose von Willebrand disease by history and interpretation of laboratory tests.

301. Answer: D

Answer: She most likely has an inhibitor to factor VIII.
Correct evaluation of a prolonged PTT is a 1:1 mix, which provides 50% of normal factor levels. If the PTT corrects, this confirms a factor deficiency that can be further determined by assaying individual factor levels. Incubation after a mixing study allows detection of antibodies (inhibitors) directed against coagulation factors. Prolongation of the PTT after initial correction is evidence for an inhibitor, which can then be titered. Specificity for the inhibitor can be determined by factor assays. In this case, the mixing study normalized the PTT and then after incubation, became prolonged again. Thus, factor deficiency is not indicated. Warfarin would result in a prolonged PT.

Board Testing Point: Interpret the findings of a mixing study and determine if an inhibitor is present.

302. Answer: E

Answer: Iron deficiency.
Megaloblastic anemia is most often related to cobalamin (Vitamin B-12) or folate deficiencies and typically demonstrates a prompt response to effective supplementation. This response, however, is capable of uncovering other coexistent deficiencies (e.g. iron deficiency) related to the increased erythroblastic activities.

This patient's reticulocyte response confirms the initial diagnosis of vitamin deficiency and the marrow's capacity to generate new red blood cells. The later shift in mean corpuscular volume (MCV), the muted reticulocyte response, and the persistent anemia are consistent with an emerging iron deficiency. Though the initial iron studies were within normal limits, they were suggestive of low body stores, which would have been depleted with an upsurge in red cell production.

B-12 deficiencies can arise secondary to absorption problems, but these are bypassed by B-12 injections. Folate absorption can be impaired by malnutrition and malabsorption, but are not consistent with the shift in the patient's MCV. Myelofibrosis is a disorder of fibrotic changes in the marrow, with red cell production abnormalities and usually with splenomegaly. The cells noted with this disorder are usually atypical including tear-drop cells and increased numbers of RBC precursor cells (myelocytes, promyelocytes), which are larger than mature RBCs. These larger cells present with an elevated MCV. A hemolytic anemia would have led to a reticulocytosis if no other deficiencies were present.

Board Testing Point: Diagnose iron deficiency anemia status post-treatment of a megaloblastic anemia.

303. Answer: B

Answer: Placement of an inferior vena cava filter.
Protein C deficiency is associated with a hypercoagulable state that tends to be recurrent. Pulmonary embolism is a life-threatening complication of deep venous thrombosis, and the risk of death is increased in the presence of pulmonary hypertension. An inferior vena cava filter can reduce risk from pulmonary embolism, but may increase long-term DVT recurrence. The patient's history of recurrent DVT and PE, cardiac status, and inability to maintain adequate anti-coagulation with warfarin makes him a serious candidate for an inferior vena cava filter. Protein C is also associated with skin necrosis in the early stages of warfarin therapy. Repetitive episodes of warfarin bolus enhance this risk and the patient's noncompliance with warfarin therapy make this option impractical for long-term therapy. Enoxaparin is expensive and requires daily compliance, which is unlikely in this scenario. Neither aspirin nor clopidogrel is effective in treating protein C deficiency.

Board Testing Point: Recommend therapy for a patient with recurrent thrombosis, pulmonary emboli and pulmonary hypertension secondary to Protein C deficiency who is nonadherent to anticoagulation therapy.

304. Answer: C

Answer: Thalassemia.
Red cell distribution width (RDW) is a measure of the range of a person's circulating red cell size. It is increased in conditions that have a variety of circulating red blood cell populations (microcytic/macrocytic cells, increased reticulocytes) or a sample with damaged red cells resulting in cells and fragments of varying size. Conditions that tend to have large variation in red cell size include iron deficiency anemia, hemolytic anemias, and spherocytosis. Red cells in patients with thalassemia have a defect in hemoglobin synthesis, but the defect tends to produce cells of uniform size, and the RDW tends to remain within the normal range.

Board Testing Point: Use the RDW to determine the etiology of an anemia.

305. Answer: E

Answer: Peripheral smear showing clumped platelets, normalization of platelet count using heparinized tube.
This patient has pseudothrombocytopenia, and her actual platelet count is normal. This may be recognized by visualizing clumps of platelets on a regular blood smear; using a heparinized (or sodium citrate) tube will give an accurate platelet count. There are no clinical signs/symptoms, and no therapy is needed. Immune thrombocytopenic purpura often has lower platelet counts, and bleeding/purpura on exam, which this patient did not have. Anti-platelet and anti-RBC antibodies (Evan syndrome) presents with immune hemolytic anemia plus thrombocytopenia. This patient does not have a review of systems or examination consistent with hemophilia or endocarditis.

Board Testing Point: Recognize pseudothrombocytopenia.

306. Answer: A

Answer: Reactive thrombocytosis.
Elevated platelet counts may be caused by autonomous increases in production (myeloproliferative disorders, myelodysplasia, leukemia) or secondary causes that stimulate the bone marrow to increase platelet production. Reactive thrombocytosis is diagnosed when no primary hematologic condition exists to account for the thrombocytosis, but when a medical condition leads to elevated platelets (inflammation, infection, chronic illness). A reactive marrow may cause extreme thrombocytosis (platelet count > 1,000,000 cells/mm^3), and may be caused by rebound after treatment of other hematologic conditions or iron deficiency anemia, as with this patient.

Essential thrombocytosis is diagnosed only when all other causes for elevated platelets are excluded and may be confirmed by bone marrow biopsy. Platelets are typically not elevated in hemoconcentrated individuals. Myelodysplasia may cause thrombocytosis, but bone marrow biopsy would be needed to confirm, and in this case, the slow bleeding is an obvious etiology. Mixed cryoglobulinemia may cause spurious or pseudothrombocytosis, but this patient's clinical picture is not consistent with cryoglobulinemia.

Board Testing Point: Recognize causes of secondary thrombocytosis.

307. Answer: A

Answer: Vitamin K supplementation and discontinuation of the cephalexin.
Although rare in patients who are not seriously ill or malnourished, antibiotics may cause coagulopathy in a number of ways; this is more common with prolonged use of antibiotics, since gut bacteria synthesize absorbable Vitamin K (menaquinone). Other causes include short bowel syndrome and a diet lacking vitamin K. ANA levels of 1:80 are often nonspecific, and this patient has none of the other criteria for lupus. Splinter hemorrhages, while seen in endocarditis, are also seen in vitamin K deficiency. Cryoprecipitate is not necessary to reverse this patient's coagulopathy, since vitamin K supplementation should correct the problem. Anticoagulation is not appropriate for this patient.

Board Testing Point: Associate clinically significant vitamin K deficiency with the use of cephalosporin antibiotics.

308. Answer: C

Answer: A bleeding time.
Her family history is very suggestive of a bleeding disorder, and Von Willebrand disease would be most the most common. Her personal history suggests that further workup is needed. A bleeding time would be the next correct step from the options listed. Remember: The hemophilias are X-linked recessive, so affected females are unusual. Antiphospholipid antibody syndrome has a prolonged PTT, but these patients clot rather than bleed. With a thrombin time test for abnormal fibrinogen, you would expect to see prolongation of the PT and PTT.

Board Testing Point: Recognize the findings of von Willebrand disease and the importance of a bleeding time study.

309. Answer: B

Answer: Plasmapheresis.
Thrombotic thrombocytopenic purpura (TTP) is a bleeding disorder caused by a decrease in ADAMTS 13 activity. ADAMTS 13 is a protease that regulates von Willebrand factor activity. The decreased activity of this protease is caused either by an inhibitor antibody or, less commonly, by an actual deficiency of ADAMTS 13. The classic symptoms associated with TTP are: hemolytic anemia with intravascular hemorrhage, fever, thrombocytopenia, decreased renal function, and neurological findings (confusion, altered mental status). A fairly crude, yet effective, memory tool for this condition is **FARTS**: Fever, microangiopathic hemolytic **A**nemia, **R**enal failure, **T**hrombocytopenia and **S**trokes/CNS disease. Treatment of this condition relies on 1) plasmapheresis to remove the inhibitory antibody, or 2) exchange transfusion using fresh frozen plasma. Immunoglobulin therapy, splenectomy, and immunosuppressive agents are treatment options for idiopathic thrombocytopenic purpura (ITP), but are not primary therapies for TTP.

Board Testing Point: Diagnose and treat thrombotic thrombocytopenic purpura.

310. Answer: B

Answer: Anemia of chronic disease.
Explanation: The iron study patterns for anemia are as follows:

	Iron	IBC	Ferritin	Soluble transferrin receptor
Iron deficiency	low	high	low	high
Anemia of chronic disease	low	low	normal/high	normal

In this case, the patient's findings are consistent with anemia of chronic disease.

Board Testing Point: Recognize the patterns of iron studies for anemia of chronic disease.

311. Answer: A

Answer: Iron deficiency anemia.
Explanation: The iron study patterns for anemia are as follows:

	Iron	IBC	Ferritin	Soluble transferrin receptor
Iron deficiency	low	high	low	high
Anemia of chronic disease	low	low	normal/high	normal

In this case, the patient's findings are consistent with iron deficiency anemia.

Board Testing Point: Recognize the iron study patterns in iron deficiency anemia.

312. Answer: A

Answer: Iron deficiency anemia
Explanation: The iron study patterns for anemia are as follows:

	Iron	IBC	Ferritin	Soluble transferrin receptor
Iron deficiency	low	high	low	high
Anemia of chronic disease	low	low	normal/high	normal

In this case, she has the findings consistent with iron deficiency anemia. Be sure you know that you expect a high soluble transferrin receptor in iron deficiency. This test has been useful in discriminating iron deficiency anemia from anemia of chronic disease.

Board Testing Point: Recognize the use of the soluble transferrin receptor in differentiating between iron deficiency anemia and anemia of chronic disease.

313. Answer: D

Answer: Hemochromatosis.
This disorder arises from abnormal storage of iron, affecting organ function in many areas. Classic characteristics include hepatomegaly, skin pigmentation, diabetes mellitus, cardiac involvement, arthritic complaints, and hypogonadism. This can occur from genetically based deficits in iron metabolism or from chronic iron overloading. The disease tends to be progressive and can lead to liver cirrhosis and congestive heart failure. Treatment is based on reducing body iron stores, and the basic interventions rely on repetitive phlebotomy.

The high serum ferritin is suggestive of the large iron stores. Hepatomegaly is a common finding but, unlike alcoholic liver disease, the liver functions are often normal. Anemia is not a direct component of hemochromatosis but can coexist if the etiology is not iron deficiency. Sideroblastic anemia exhibits difficulty in management of iron within red blood cells but not in general tissues. Repetitive transfusions for sideroblastic anemia, and similar processes such as thalassemia, are an iatrogenic risk for developing secondary hemochromatosis. Polycythemia vera presents as increased level of circulating red blood cells, not increased iron, and is distinguished by an increased red cell mass index.

Board Testing Point: Recognize the clinical and laboratory findings of hemochromatosis.

---

314. Answer: B

Answer: M3 AML with a t(15,17).
Association of acute leukemia subtypes with clinical syndromes is helpful in making a diagnosis. M3 with t(15, 17), also known as acute promyelocytic leukemia, is commonly associated with DIC. Acute monocytic leukemia is known for its association with subcutaneous skin nodules and gum hypertrophy.

Board Testing Point: Associate M3 AML with a translocation of chromosomes 15 and 17 (acute promyelocytic leukemia) and disseminated intravascular coagulation.

---

315. Answer: A

Answer: Desmopressin.
von Willebrand factor functions as a carrier for factor VIII and facilitates platelet adhesion during clotting. Two recognized therapies are factor VIII concentrate infusions, which include significant levels of von Willebrand factor, and desmopressin. Previous concerns over the potential for HIV transmission have been improved with current preparations of factor VIII concentrate. This option, however, is not inexpensive and requires administration. Desmopressin is significantly less expensive and successfully controls bleeding in oral procedures for many patients with von Willebrand disease. It is not effective for all individuals, and response should be tested prior to therapeutic use. von Willebrand disease is not an inflammatory process, and steroids have no effect. The bleeding disorder is not secondary to defective platelets, and platelet infusions likewise have no effect. EACA (ε-aminocaproic acid) is an effective potent anti-fibrinolytic agent for oral procedures, but is more commonly used as an adjunct in hemophiliac patients.

Board Testing Point: Prescribe desmopressin before a dental procedure in a patient with von Willebrand disease.

---

316. Answer: A

Answer: Bone marrow aspirate, biopsy, and cytogenetic analysis.
This patient most likely has essential thrombocytosis with elevation of all of her blood counts and no clear reason to have secondary elevation (most common is iron deficiency anemia, and her indices and hematocrit are normal). Her symptoms at present have resolved, but will weigh in the decision to treat her. She does need cytogenetic analysis to rule out other myeloproliferative disorders such as CML; thus, marrow with cytogenetics is your best possible choice. Ferritin level is not helpful, and platelet pheresis is not indicated.

Board Testing Point: Recognize the findings of essential thrombocytosis and its appropriate workup.

---

317. Answer: D

Answer: Thrombotic thrombocytopenic purpura.
She has the classic pentad found in thrombotic thrombocytopenic purpura (TTP). This includes severe thrombocytopenia, microangiopathic hemolytic anemia (schistocytes also known as "helmet cells," as depicted in the peripheral smear), fluctuating neurologic signs (especially confusion), renal failure, and fever. Petechiae are

also common. The normal PT and PTT found in TTP help differentiate it from DIC. The treatment of choice for TTP is plasmapheresis. If not available, then IVIG may be given.

Hemolytic uremic syndrome is similar to TTP clinically and pathologically, except that HUS mainly affects the afferent arterioles and glomeruli of the kidney and usually occurs in children.

Idiopathic thrombocytopenic purpura (ITP) is usually of a chronic and relapsing course in adults. ITP causes thrombocytopenia but does not cause any of the other findings associated with TTP. There are no other hematologic abnormalities or renal involvement with ITP.

Glanzmann thrombasthenia is due to a low glycoprotein IIB-IIIa complex and results in bleeding as fibrinogen is unable to cross-connect. It has a normal platelet count.

Board Testing Point: Recognize the pentad of TTP.

318. Answer: B

Answer: Vitamin B-12 deficiency.
The peripheral smear is showing you a very hypersegmented neutrophil. Note also that the RBC is pretty large compared to the neutrophil, making it likely macrocytic as well. Of the choices, only Vitamin B-12 deficiency would give you a macrocytic RBC with a hypersegmented neutrophil. Folate deficiency would also give you a macrocytic anemia with hypersegmented neutrophils. Iron deficiency anemia would present with microcytosis. With TTP, you would look for schistocytes or RBC fragments. ITP would present with bleeding diathesis or low platelets. ALL would present with blast cells in a much younger individual.

Board Testing Point: Recognize that hypersegmented neutrophils are associated with vitamin B-12 deficiency (and folate deficiency).

319. Answer: B

Answer: Burr cells (echinocytes).
A burr cell is an RBC with multiple small projections distributed across its surface. The projections tend to be dispersed evenly, have blunt ends, and are uniform in size. These characteristics help differentiate burr cells from spur cells (acanthocytes), which feature a small number of irregularly spaced and sized, thorn-like projections. Burr cells are often an artifact related to storage or an elevated pH level, but they can also be indicative of a variety of diseases and conditions, including uremia, pyruvate kinase deficiency, lymphosarcoma, glomerulonephritis, and peptic ulcers. The reason for their development is not fully understood; however, it is likely that acid-base and electrolyte disturbances associated with uremia and glomerulonephritis may play a role in the development of burr cells.

Board Testing Point: Recognize Burr cells in the setting of uremia.

320. Answer: C

Answer: Hereditary elliptocytosis.
Hereditary elliptocytosis is a congenital hemolytic disorder characterized by RBCs that are either elongated (cigar- or oval-shaped) or show irregular degrees of poikilocytosis. It results because of a defect in one of the skeletal proteins in the RBC membrane. It is estimated that hereditary elliptocytosis occurs in between 1/2000 and 1/5000. Most individuals affected are asymptomatic and do not require any therapy. It is autosomal dominant in

inheritance with at least 4 genetic loci involved in the pathogenesis. Heterozygotes (common hereditary elliptocytosis) are almost always asymptomatic. Homozygotes usually have severe hemolytic anemia and are classified as having hereditary pyropoikilocytosis.

Diagnosis is made by finding the classic elliptocytes on peripheral smear. Elliptocytes can be seen in other diseases, such as megaloblastic and iron-deficiency anemia, but are associated with the other findings of those diseases (anemia, etc.) and make up less than 25% of the RBCs, as compared to hereditary elliptocytosis causing > 25% elliptocytes. An increased reticulocyte count is common (up to 4%). Thalassemia trait would not result in this finding, and sickle cell disease would present with classic sickle cells and be symptomatic. Vitamin B-12 deficiency would result in hypersegmentation of neutrophils and RBC macrocytosis.

Board Testing Point: Recognize elliptocytes and their benign nature in heterozygotes with hereditary elliptocytosis.

321. Answer: D

Answer: Sickle cell.
This is a classic sickle cell. Be able to identify it on the examination. Helmet cells and schistocytes are just different names for the same cell (helmet-shaped). Elliptocytes are cigar- or oval-shaped. Plasma cells are mature B-cell lymphocytes and not red cells at all.

Board Testing Point: Recognize a sickle cell in a peripheral smear.

322. Answer: E

Answer: All of the options are associated with this type of cell.
This is a plasma cell, which is a mature B lymphocyte specialized for producing immunoglobulin. They are rarely found in the peripheral blood; if they are noted, then any of the choices could be associated with an increased number of peripheral blood plasma cells.

Board Testing Point: Recognize the association of a peripheral blood plasma cell with multiple myeloma, Waldenström's macroglobulinemia, MGUS, or plasma cell leukemia.

323. Answer: E

Answer: Spherocyte.
Spherocytosis is usually an autosomal dominant (75%; 25% are autosomal recessive) red blood cell disorder seen mainly in those of Northern European ancestry. The incidence is about 1/5000. About 25% of cases are due to new mutations. Spherocytosis results in a hemolytic anemia due to lysis as they pass through the spleen. Four abnormalities in red cell membrane proteins have been recognized: 1) isolated spectrin deficiency, 2) combined spectrin and ankyrin deficiency, 3) band 3 deficiency, and 4) protein 4.2 defects. 60-75% of patients have moderate disease with mild-to-moderate anemia, splenomegaly, and intermittent jaundice. 20-30% of those affected are generally asymptomatic. Splenectomy is indicated for severe disease and those with refractory anemias.

Board Testing Point: Recognize a spherocyte on peripheral smear.

324. Answer: C

Answer: Splenectomy.
This smear is showing you Howell-Jolly bodies. These occur usually after splenectomy. Howell-Jolly bodies are the result of fragmentation of the RBC nucleus (karyorrhexis) causing the formation of small black "pellets." This occurs normally, and the spleen efficiently removes them; however, without a functional spleen these remain on the surface of the RBCs.

Board Testing Point: Recognize Howell-Jolly bodies on peripheral smear.

325. Answer: A

Answer: Thalassemia.
Teardrop red blood cells are found in thalassemia, myelofibrosis and other myeloproliferative disorders, pernicious anemia, and myeloid metaplasia.

Board Testing Point: Recognize teardrop RBCs on peripheral smear and know their disease associations.

326. Answer: A

Answer: Parvovirus B19 infection.
Infection with Parvovirus B19 causes transient aplastic crisis patients with hemoglobinopathies and is consistent with the findings of severe anemia and reticulocytopenia. The transient arrest of erythropoiesis results in a sudden fall in hemoglobin concentrations in individuals with, for example, sickle cell disease and thalassemia. Patients with sickle cell disease are at increased risk of infection with *Salmonella* and pneumococcal organisms, but the vignette does not describe a febrile, toxic patient with septicemia. These patients are also at increased risk for vaso-occlusive events such as pulmonary infarction and stroke, but the clinical scenario described in the question is not consistent with either of these complications.

Board Testing Point: Recognize parvovirus B-19 as an etiology of aplastic crisis in patients with sickle cell disease.

327. Answer: A

Answer: Hepatic venography.
He most likely has polycythemia rubra vera with the presence of primary erythrocytosis with organomegaly. A complication of this disorder is hypercoagulability, with hepatic vein thrombosis being a particular problem seen. Hepatic vein thrombosis would lead to Budd-Chiari syndrome where you would have a grossly enlarged liver with severe ascites. The best way to diagnosis this is by hepatic venography or liver biopsy where you would look for sinusoidal dilatation. The other choices would not be diagnostic because you really need to see the architecture of the sinusoids to make the diagnosis.

Board Testing Point: Recognize polycythemia rubra vera and the risk of hepatic vein thrombosis.

328. Answer: D

Answer: B-12 deficiency.
This patient has Zollinger-Ellison syndrome, which is managed through the use of high-dose proton pump inhibitors. High doses of proton pump inhibitors can decrease absorption of vitamin B-12. Oral B-12 absorption is reduced by 90% in volunteers taking 40 mg of omeprazole. Folate deficiency could cause the elevated MCV, but high-dose proton pump inhibitors do not affect folate levels. Alcohol is much less likely. Lead deficiency and sideroblastic anemia would not have an elevated MCV.

Board Testing Point: Recognize the association of high-dose proton pump inhibitor use and possible B-12 deficiency.

ONCOLOGY

329. Answer: C

Answer: Bronchoalveolar carcinoma.
Bronchoalveolar carcinoma is a subtype of adenocarcinoma. Although smoking is still the most common risk factor for all types of lung cancer, lung cancers in younger patients tend to occur more commonly in women and are more likely to be adenocarcinomas (also the most common lung cancer in non-smokers). As the name implies, bronchoalveolar carcinoma may appear as an alveolar filling process, and may be mistaken for pneumonia or congestive heart failure (although it more commonly presents as a nodule or mass in an asymptomatic patient). "Bronchorrhea," the production of copious, watery sputum (> 100 mL/day), may be seen in bronchoalveolar carcinoma (as well as chronic bronchitis, panbronchiolitis, and bronchiectasis). The longer duration of symptoms, lack of response to antibiotics, presence of "B" symptoms and physical findings in this patient make the diagnoses of pneumonia and CHF much less likely. Idiopathic pulmonary fibrosis usually presents in older individuals, has a longer duration of symptoms (12-18 months), and has a different appearance on CXR. This patient has no risks for *Pneumocystis jiroveci* pneumonia, which usually presents as an insidious pneumonia in HIV or other immunocompromised patients and rarely causes pleural effusions.

Board Testing Point: Recognize bronchoalveolar carcinoma in a non-smoking patient.

330. Answer: B

Answer: Bleomycin.
Most anti-cancer therapies have significant negative side effects, especially harmful on rapidly regenerating tissues. These include nausea and vomiting, hair loss, mucosal ulcers, and bone marrow compromise. Individual chemotherapeutic agents may also have more specific side effects. For example, doxorubicin is associated with cardiac damage, vincristine with peripheral neuropathies, and dacarbazine with a metallic taste. Bleomycin's activity is enhanced by increased oxygen tension levels, but the high tension can cause increased damage in pulmonary tissues. Pulmonary inflammation occurs in approximately 10% of patients receiving bleomycin.

Board Testing Point: Review the chemotherapy agents and their common side-effects.

331. Answer: C

Answer: Urine cytology, abdominal CT to rule out an abdominal malignancy.
This patient likely has renal cell carcinoma (RCC). Signs/symptoms of renal cell carcinoma: abdominal pain, hematuria, abdominal mass (may be difficult to palpate in overweight individuals). 11% have scrotal varicoceles, so have a high suspicion for RCC if the varicocele does not empty with recumbency (implying gonadal vein obstruction). These patients may also have malignancy-associated thromboembolism (portal vein, Budd-Chiari's, PE, or migrating IVC clot). In addition, 1-5% of patients with RCC have significant erythrocytosis because of increases in erythropoietin production. Imaging: CT is best; ultrasound/MRI may also be helpful. Phlebotomy is not necessary at this time; the erythrocytosis should improve after resection. Bone marrow biopsy would be warranted for suspicion of a primary hematologic disorder; this patient's erythrocytosis is secondary. Testicular evaluation for carcinoma should be performed in patients with a testicular mass. Fertility counseling is not indicated. Doxorubicin would cause cardiac toxicity.

Board Testing Point: Associate renal cell carcinoma with secondary erythrocytosis.

332. Answer: B

Answer: *Helicobacter pylori* (*H. pylori*).
Infectious agents have been linked with several disease processes. *H. pylori* has been associated with the development of gastric MALT lymphomas. The connection is evidenced by the fact that the majority of MALT lymphomas of the gastric mucosa resolve when *H. pylori* is eradicated. EBV is linked with several other lymphomas, including Burkitt's. *Tropheryma whipplei* is the causative agent of Whipple disease, an insidious disease of the bowels and central nervous system ("diarrhea and dementia"). Human herpes virus 8 is associated with a systemic diffuse lymphadenopathy, Castleman disease. Hepatitis B raises the risk of hepatocellular carcinoma in patients who develop cirrhosis as a result of the viral infection.

Board Testing Point: Associate *H. pylori* with the development of gastric MALT lymphoma and recognize that eradication of *H. pylori* may treat the underlying tumor.

333. Answer: C

Answer: Colposcopy.
HPV has been strongly associated with the development of cervical cancer. The virus exhibits both high- and low-risk serotypes; types 16 and 18 are the most important and are considered the "high-risk" HPV types. Patients infected with high-risk variants require close supervision, and most guidelines recommend direct follow-up with colposcopy. In this patient, where follow-up is not certain, colposcopic examination is the most appropriate recommendation.

One-year follow-up might be appropriate if the HPV variant were a low-risk subtype. Follow-up in 3-6 months is most appropriate in a patient with inflammatory changes on Pap smear, but negative HPV status. Acetic acid applications may help highlight areas of viral involvement but are not therapeutic for the infection. Podophyllin for HPV without visible lesions is not indicated.

Board Testing Point: Recognize colposcopy as the next step in evaluation of ASCUS.

334. Answer: A

Answer: Osteogenic sarcoma.
Retinoblastoma is an aggressive neoplastic process involving the retina of young children. Left untreated, this neoplasm is typically fatal. Former intervention was typically enucleation. More recently, external beam radiation therapy, "Brady therapy," cryotherapy, laser therapy, and chemotherapy have been added to the therapeutic options. Retinoblastomas occur through a hereditary or non-hereditary fashion. Bilateral retinoblastomas are always of the hereditary form and are associated with an increased risk for osteogenic sarcomas, soft tissue sarcomas, and malignant melanoma. These secondary tumors often occur decades after the initial presentation. The use of radiation therapy can also increase the risk of secondary neoplasms. Incidence of Ewing sarcoma, multiple myeloma, and parathyroid tumors are not increased in patients with a history of retinoblastoma.

Board Testing Point: Recognize that it may take decades for a secondary tumor to occur after successful treatment of childhood retinoblastoma.

335. Answer: B

Answer: Pretreatment with oral allopurinol.
Burkitt lymphoma presents in three situations: endemic (primarily in Africa), sporadic, and associated with immunodeficiency (HIV). Treatment of Burkitt's has a tendency to precipitate tumor lysis syndrome, a surge in metabolic wastes and electrolyte shifts driven by rapid cell destruction that is often caused by chemotherapy. Principal characteristics include hyperkalemia, hyperphosphatemia (with calcium precipitation and hypocalcemia), and hyperuricemia with uric acid deposition in the renal parenchyma leading to decreased renal function. Allopurinol therapy can help mitigate renal damage and should be considered in patients with Burkitt lymphoma, acute lymphocytic leukemia, and other high-bulk, non-solid tumors. Steroids do not prevent the uric acid effects and may actually precipitate cell lysis. Calcium is not the cause of the pathology but a result of hyperphosphatemia, and calcium supplements may lead to increased precipitation. An alkaline pH can reduce damage. Acidification would be contraindicated. Hydration, allopurinol, and alkalinization are the standard interventions, and dialysis may be required for severe or progressive cases.

Board Testing Point: Pretreatment of Burkitt lymphoma with allopurinol is necessary to prevent tumor-lysis syndrome.

336. Answer: D

Answer: Germ cell tumor.
A painless testicular mass in a young adult should always raise the possibility of testicular neoplasm. A history of undescended testicle increases the risk of malignant degeneration. A varicocele typically presents like a "bag of worms" and is normally left-sided or bilateral because of venous flow patterns. Unilateral right-sided varicoceles are very uncommon. Spermatoceles are found on the superior pole of the testis and can normally be palpated separately from the testis. Hydroceles are fluid-filled and may range from firm to spongy. Hydroceles transilluminate well.

Board Testing Point: Recognize the presentation of testicular cancer.

337. Answer: B

Answer: Lymph node involvement of the spleen, splenic hilar nodes, and celiac nodes.
Prognosis for non-Hodgkin lymphoma can be based on the International Prognostic Index. The factors used in this rating system are based on age, Ann Arbor staging for Hodgkin lymphoma, lactate dehydrogenase (LDH), extranodal lymphoma involvement, and life function performance status. Age older than 60, elevated LDH, Ann Arbor staging assignment of III or IV, more than 1 extranodal site of involvement, or diminished life function score have a worse prognosis. Under the Ann Arbor staging system, involvement that crosses the diaphragm (mediastinum and abdominal para-aortic nodes) is worse prognostically than involvement restricted to one side of the diaphragm (the spleen, splenic hilar nodes and celiac nodes). Bone marrow involvement is also an indicator of worse prognosis. Due to the variable outcomes of different subtypes of lymphoma, the risk assignment and prognosis vary. Diffuse large cell lymphoma tends to have a more aggressive course, while follicular and small lymphocytic lymphomas tend to have a better prognosis.

Board Testing Point: Identify prognostic indicators in non-Hodgkin lymphoma.

338. Answer: B

Answer: Mammogram and clinical breast exam starting now.
Women whose first-degree relatives have been diagnosed with early-age breast cancer should have early screening with mammogram and clinical breast examination. Typically, screening should start 5 years prior to the earliest diagnosed case of cancer.

Testing should be considered for BRCA1 and BRCA2 hormones that are associated with early-age familial breast cancer. P53 mutations are associated with many types of malignancies, and the Lynch II syndrome is associated with hereditary non-polyposis colorectal cancer (HNPCC) and increased risk of ovarian cancer. Bilateral oophorectomy is not recommended for prophylaxis of breast cancer.

Board Testing Point: Evaluate risk factors for breast cancer and determine when screening should be initiated.

339. Answer: D

Answer: Treatment should include CNS prophylaxis.
Burkitt lymphoma is an unusual subtype of non-Hodgkin lymphoma with both endemic (African form) and sporadic presentations. The sporadic form is typically seen in the United States and consists of a rapidly enlarging abdominal mass. Burkitt's is considered a very aggressive subtype of B-cell lymphoma and is exquisitely sensitive to chemotherapy if the disease is found early. The treatment regimen should always include CNS prophylaxis, since involvement/relapse at this site is common.

Board Testing Point: Design a treatment regimen for Burkitt lymphoma and include the CNS.

340. Answer: E

Answer: Lumpectomy and radiation therapy followed by adjuvant tamoxifen.
Definitive therapy for this patient could include both lumpectomy with radiation therapy or modified radical mastectomy, both of which historically provide the same results. This patient's tumor is small enough for either maneuver to provide primary tumor control. Combination chemotherapy is not required, but due to the size of the tumor (3 cm), adjuvant therapy (tamoxifen) is indicated. Nodal status is unknown, thus assumed negative; and hormone receptors are positive, allowing the use of hormonal therapy alone as adjuvant treatment.

Board Testing Point: Determine appropriate therapy for a patient with breast cancer.

341. Answer: E

Answer: Inguinal orchiectomy with appropriate CT scans for staging.
With an asymptomatic mass this size, malignancy is likely; thus, primary surgery rather than observation is the treatment of choice. An inguinal approach is appropriate with further treatment dictated by the stage of the disease. Chemotherapy should be given only after a diagnosis is established. Treatment with antibiotics can be done initially, although the size and lack of associated symptoms would discourage this approach. Transscrotal biopsy is contraindicated because of the risk of tumor spread.

Board Testing Point: Recognize the appropriate management for a patient with an enlarging testicular mass.

342. Answer: A

Answer: Counsel him that his original pathology results were incorrect.
Seminomas are never associated with AFP; thus, this pathologic diagnosis must be incorrect. Knowing the half-life for these markers is useful for assessing response to treatment. AFP has a half-life of about 5 days and BHCG about 24 hours; suspect persistent disease when the markers remain elevated. Once therapy is complete, he must be followed more closely than every 6 months. Further treatment must be defined by disease after surgery but would not include bone marrow transplantation or retroperitoneal radiation as initial treatment.

Board Testing Point: Recognize the laboratory findings that distinguish between seminomas and non-seminomas.

343. Answer: D

Answer: Emergent leukophoresis.
There are several steps needed in the workup, including a bone marrow aspirate and cytogenetics. However, with a blast count of > 100,000, emergent leukophoresis should be done while the evaluation is ongoing. This is a question that makes you address the most urgent problem, the markedly elevated WBC blast count.

Board Testing Point: Recognize the importance of emergent leukophoresis in the setting of an extremely high WBC blast count.

344. Answer: C

Answer: Squamous cell lung cancer.
This patient has hypercalcemia with symptoms of dehydration associated with a central lung mass. The corrected calcium level (adjusted for the low albumin) is 12.40 mg/dL.
Paraneoplastic syndromes are commonly associated with the pulmonary neoplasms:
Squamous cell carcinomas: central, cavitary, hypercalcemia;
Small cell carcinomas: central, neuroendocrine, SIADH, dermatomyositis;
Large cell carcinomas: peripheral, scar carcinomas;
Bronchoalveolar adenocarcinoma is not associated with smoking.

Be familiar with these associations!

Board Testing Point: Interpret laboratory tests and identify hypercalcemia; associate hypercalcemia with squamous cell cancer in patients with lung masses

345. Answer: B

Answer: Bronchoalveolar cancer (BAC).
The tumor in this case is diffuse and involving the entire middle lobe, but several separate lesions are not visible as is common in metastatic lesions. He has been symptomatic for an extended period of time, making CAP unlikely. Additionally, he is afebrile and has no shortness of breath, as is commonly associated with CAP. Metastatic melanoma presenting in this fashion would be very unusual. Lung cancer is divided into two major categories: small cell and non-small cell. Sub-types of non-small cell lung cancers include: squamous cell, large cell and adenocarcinoma. Bronchoalveolar lung cancer is a type of adenocarcinoma. Adenocarcinomas, specifically of bronchoalveolar type, have the weakest association with smoking cigarettes. Approximately 1/3 of

patients with BAC have never smoked. BAC also demonstrates unusual radiographic presentations, often resembling pneumonia. Paraneoplastic syndromes are commonly associated with the pulmonary neoplasms:

Squamous cell carcinomas: central, cavitary, hypercalcemia;

Small cell carcinomas: central, neuroendocrine, SIADH, dermatomyositis;

Large cell carcinomas: peripheral, scar carcinomas;

Bronchoalveolar adenocarcinoma is not associated with smoking.

Be familiar with these associations!

Board Testing Point: Identify a chronic illness based on history; associate BAC with diffuse consolidation on a chest radiograph, and recognize there is a lack of association with smoking with this pathology.

346. Answer: A

Answer: Squamous cell lung cancer.

This is a case of a cavitating lung mass. The differential diagnosis of lung masses that cavitate is long and includes: lung abscesses, tuberculosis, septic emboli, rheumatoid nodules, Wegener's granulomatosis, blastomycosis, nocardiosis, squamous cell lung cancer, and rarely, *Pneumocystis* pneumonia. To narrow down the list of possibilities, you will want to consider the epidemiologic risk factors associated with each etiology. For example, septic emboli causing cavitating lung masses occur most prominently in patients with staphylococcal bacteremia. So, you want to look for recurrent furunculosis or injection drug use in the history. The history provided specifically excludes blastomycosis by telling you that the patient does not hunt and has not traveled to wooded areas. Because he is a long-time, heavy smoker, his risk of cancer exceeds his risk of blastomycosis. Recall these factoids about lung cancers:

Squamous cell carcinomas: central, cavitary;

Small cell carcinomas: central, neuroendocrine, SIADH, dermatomyositis;

Large cell carcinomas: peripheral, scar carcinomas;

Bronchoalveolar not associated with smoking.

Be familiar with these associations!

Board Testing Point: Identify the most likely etiology of a cavitating lung mass in a smoker.

347. Answer: E

Answer: CT scan and biopsy of any identifiable mass.

Superior vena cave syndrome is an oncologic emergency. Definitive treatment will depend upon the cause of the obstruction; thus, biopsy should be pursued prior to treatment. Several malignancies would best be treated with chemotherapy while others would require primary radiation therapy. Biopsy is the best answer to define the diagnosis and then determine possible therapy.

Board Testing Point: Recognize the superior vena cava syndrome and the appropriate test to perform if it is suspected.

348. Answer: D

Answer: Dexamethasone intravenously, emergent spine MRI.
This patient's clinical history is entirely consistent with spinal cord compression from metastatic disease. Common malignancies that metastasize to bone include breast, lung, and prostate cancer; but renal cell cancer, thyroid cancer, and melanoma also spread to bone. Pain is the most common symptom, but later progresses to weakness, a sensory level, incoordination and incontinence. Patients with impending cord compression should receive immediate corticosteroids and neuroimaging. Further treatment will be dictated by the location and type of compression, as well as the type of malignancy; however, prompt neurosurgical and oncologic intervention is paramount. X-rays of the spine, while possibly identifying bony metastases, would not be sufficient to diagnose cord compression. Elective evaluation by orthopaedics or neurology would not be appropriate because waiting for their involvement would likely delay diagnostics and treatment. While spinal stenosis may present with back pain or pseudoclaudication, this patient's cancer history and progressive symptoms, as well as the abnormal neurologic exam, are worrisome for spinal metastases and require prompt evaluation and management.

Board Testing Point: Recognize the clinical features of spinal cord compression from epidural metastasis.

349. Answer: C

Answer: Vincristine.
Most anti-cancer therapies have significant side effects, particularly on rapidly regenerating tissues. These include nausea and vomiting, hair loss, mucosal ulcers, and bone marrow compromise. Individual chemotherapeutic agents may also have additional specific side effects. For example, doxorubicin is associated with cardiac damage, Bleomycin with damage to pulmonary tissues and inflammation, and dacarbazine with a metallic taste. Vincristine is most notably associated with peripheral neuropathies.

Board Testing Point: Know the side effects of commonly used chemotherapeutic agents.

350. Answer: C

Answer: A thyroid panel.
A very common complication of radiation therapy for patients with Hodgkin disease is hypothyroidism, which her symptoms support. There is no indication to look for low calcium or perform pulmonary function tests. Repeat CT scan is unnecessary. You should also be on the lookout for early coronary artery disease since CAD is accelerated in patients who receive radiation to the chest.

Board Testing Point: Recognize the side effects of mantle radiation therapy.

351. Answer: B

Answer: Chronic myelogenous leukemia (CML).
A simple "fact" question, but an easy "gimme" question nonetheless. ☺ It will likely be on the Board exam somewhere. CML is associated with the translocation of chromosome 9 and 22. Other simple facts to remember: AML is associated with Auer rods on a bone marrow aspirate, and Hodgkin disease is associated with Reed-Sternberg cells. Non-Hodgkin lymphoma and CLL are not associated with the translocation of chromosome 9 and 22.

Board Testing Point: Associate CML with t(9,22).

352. Answer: B

Answer: Acute myelogenous leukemia (AML).
These are Auer Rods. A simple "fact" question that you may have to recognize without clinical history. Auer rods are associated only with AML. Other simple facts to know: CML is associated with translocation of chromosome 9 and 22, and Hodgkin disease is associated with Reed-Sternberg cells.

Board Testing Point: Recognize Auer rods on a bone marrow aspirate.

353. Answer: E

Answer: Cisplatin.
Cisplatin is the only agent listed that is cleared by the kidneys; and thus, its primary toxicity is renal damage. Magnesium-wasting is common. Hydration can be helpful in preventing this from occurring. Doxorubicin is most commonly associated with cardiomyopathy. Methotrexate causes mucositis and diarrhea. Vincristine causes neurotoxicity (peripheral neuropathy). Vinblastine causes myelotoxicity.

Board Testing Point: Identify side effects for common chemotherapeutic agents.

354. Answer: D

Answer: Endometrial cancer.
Hormonal replacement therapy (HRT) in the post- or peri-menopausal patient has become a more complicated issue after the recognition of serious complications associated with its use. The Women's Health Initiative (WHI), scheduled to be completed in 2005, was discontinued early in 2004 because of the observed increased risk of heart disease, stroke, venous thromboembolism and breast cancer over a 5 year follow-up in women taking combined estrogen/progestin replacement. WHI also sponsored an unopposed estrogen versus placebo trial in women who had undergone hysterectomy and did not require the progestin in their replacement regimen. This trial was also discontinued early, but there was no increase in cardiac events or breast cancer; however, stroke and venous thromboembolism was also increased in this group. In both groups, the risk of fracture was decreased. Data from the HERS trials I and II confirmed that combination replacement with estrogen/progestin confers NO cardiac protection. As a result, the current position statement from the North American Menopause Society states that the only indication for estrogen replacement (either combined or unopposed) in our current climate is to ameliorate menopausal symptoms. Regardless of why the estrogens are prescribed, unopposed estrogen therapy causes endometrial hyperplasia; and in some patients, cancer has occurred less than 6 months after initiating unopposed estrogen treatments. Therefore, unopposed estrogens should never be used except in women who have had hysterectomies.

Board Testing Point: Associate unopposed estrogens with endometrial hyperplasia and development of malignancy.

355. Answer: A

Answer: Small cell lung cancer.
Hypotonic hyponatremia found in a patient with an obvious lung mass is most likely going to be caused by small cell lung cancer. Paraneoplastic syndromes are commonly associated with the pulmonary neoplasms:

Squamous cell carcinomas: central, cavitary, hypercalcemia
Small cell carcinomas: central, neuroendocrine, SIADH, dermatomyositis
Large cell carcinomas: peripheral, scar carcinomas
Bronchoalveolar not associated with smoking.

Be familiar with these associations!

Board Testing Point: Interpret serum chemistries and diagnose hypotonic hyponatremia; identify SIADH as the most common etiology of hyponatremia in patients with a lung mass.

356. Answer: E

Answer: A bone marrow aspirate and biopsy.
This patient has an elevated globulin fraction of 6 g/dL and, by serum protein electrophoresis, a small monoclonal peak. Workup for myeloma should be pursued with a marrow aspirate and biopsy and bone survey (not bone scan). Repeat SPE and UPE in 6 months are not indicated until the bone marrow aspirate and biopsy are performed. At this point, he has no indication for therapy, since his CBC is normal, as is his calcium; so follow-up rather than treatment with either chemotherapy or a bisphosphonate would be appropriate.

Board Testing Point: Recognize the findings and appropriate workup of a patient with suspected multiple myeloma.

357. Answer: E

Answer: Core biopsy.
Any palpable mass that is not cystic by ultrasound should be biopsied. Not all malignancies are associated with mammographic changes and, in particular, lobular carcinoma in situ commonly has no mammographic evidence. Testing for genetic mutations without a diagnosis is not indicated. There is no cyst present to aspirate.

Board Testing Point: Determine the next step in evaluation of a breast mass.

358. Answer: D

Answer: Osteoid osteoma.
This is a small benign tumor that is very painful, especially at night. The pain is typically relieved by aspirin only. Radiographs are distinctive as described. Osteochondromas arise from the metaphysis of long bones and present as a bony painless mass. Ewing sarcoma presents radiographically as periosteal elevation ("onion skinning"), while osteosarcoma appears as a mixed lytic and blastic ("starburst") process. Fibrous dysplasia is characterized by congenital fibrous replacement of cancellous bone.

Board Testing Point: Diagnose osteoid osteoma based on radiographic findings.

359. Answer: C

Answer: Perform a testicular exam since he is at increased risk of malignancy; the orchiopexy performed when he was a young child did not reduce the risk associated with undescended testes.
Orchiopexy improves fertility but does not alter the risk of malignancy. Most often, malignancy is due to a seminoma and can occur in either testicle, including a descended contralateral testes. Most undescended testicles are in the inguinal canal. Treatment should occur by 9-15 months of age.

Board Testing Point: Recognize that adults with a prior undescended testis are at increased risk for malignancy in their contralateral descended testicle and should be screened often.

360. Answer: C

Answer: Lymphoma and leukemia.
Wiskott-Aldrich syndrome is an X-linked recessive syndrome characterized by thrombocytopenia, atopic dermatitis, and recurrent infections. Infection with bacteria having polysaccharide capsules (e.g. *Streptococcus pneumoniae*) and EBV-associated malignancy make survival beyond adolescence rare. Renal cell carcinoma, melanoma and seminoma are not associated with this syndrome. Hepatic carcinoma is not an associated malignancy.

Board Testing Point: Recognize the malignancies associated with Wiskott-Aldrich syndrome.

361. Answer: D

Answer: Human Papillomavirus (HPV) infection is a causative agent of cervical cancer.
Cervical cancer is unique in that no other human cancer has yet to be shown to have such a clearly identified cause. HPV 16 is found in 50-60% of cervical cancers while HPV 18 is found in an additional 10-15% of cases. HPV infection is seen in 80% of women by the time they reach 50 years of age. About 60% of CIN1 cases regress while 30% persist and 10% progress to high-grade dysplasia. Only about 1% of CIN1 cases progress to invasive cervical cancer. Herpes does not cause CIN1. Many cases of HPV are asymptomatic.

Board Testing Point: Recognize Human Papillomavirus as a cause of cervical carcinoma.

362. Answer: B

Answer: African-American men and those men with a family history of prostate cancer should have screening discussion between ages 40 and 45.
Prostate cancer screening is difficult to tease out. Recommendations vary and scientific evidence to support screening programs is lacking. However, based on current practice guidelines, screening should be discussed with men beginning at age 50, although not with men over age 50 who have a comorbidity that limits their life expectancy to less than 10 years. African-American men and men with a family history of prostate cancer should have their first discussion about screening between the ages of 40 and 45. Notice that the word "discuss" is used. Guidelines state only that discussion should be initiated, not that actual screening should occur. When a decision is made to screen for prostate cancer, best evidence supports the use of a digital examination and a PSA level.

Board Testing Point: Evaluate when prostate cancer discussion should be initiated.

NEUROLOGY

363. Answer: E

Answer: CNS tumor (right hemisphere).
Of the options given, only ketoacidosis, pseudotumor cerebri, hypercalcemia, and CNS tumor can cause coma. The patient has upper motor neuron signs (hyperreflexia and spasticity), which suggest pyramidal (long-tract) involvement in the right hemisphere. The enlarged right pupil, often referred to as a "blown pupil," is caused by pressure that is directly placed on the third cranial nerve due to uncal herniation. These dramatic signs implicating a space-occupying lesion are not caused by hypercalcemia or ketoacidosis. The normal anion gap excludes ketoacidosis as an etiology.

90% of cases of pseudotumor cerebri occur in young, obese women. It is thought to be due to increased estrogens (it has been associated with the use of oral contraceptives); however, the list of possible causes is quite long. It is unusual, however, to see upper motor neuron impairment with pseudotumor. The most common presenting symptoms are usually headache and vision disturbances.

Normal pressure hydrocephalus occurs more often in older adults. It presents with the triad of ataxia, urinary incontinence, and dementia, which this patient did not demonstrate. The cause is not known, although many have proposed that it is due to an abnormality in cerebrospinal fluid production or reabsorption.

Board Testing Point: Differentiate the etiologies for neurologic findings involving cranial nerve dysfunction and upper motor neuron signs.

364. Answer: A

Answer: Chlordiazepoxide.
Patients with alcohol dependence can experience alcohol withdrawal during periods of abstinence such as a hospitalization. Due to the high prevalence of alcohol-related disease and the frequency of underreporting of alcohol consumption, many individuals at risk may go unrecognized. Among the differential diagnoses for acute delirium is alcohol withdrawal. Appropriate evaluation for serious conditions such as intracranial bleeding, respiratory abnormalities, electrolyte disturbances, and infectious causes must also be pursued.

This patient's labs are consistent with, but not diagnostic of, alcohol abuse, including elevated levels of SGOT, SGPT, GGT, and uric acid levels. The autonomic findings (including heart rate, respiratory rate, blood pressure, temperature, and agitation) are suggestive of significant alcohol withdrawal. Interventions should not await the development of seizures with delirium tremens. The most appropriate intervention for this condition is usually benzodiazepines. Anti-convulsants are generally too slow and do not alleviate the fundamental abnormality. Naloxone and clonidine have no direct role in the treatment, and antipsychotics are both unnecessary and inappropriate.

Board Testing Point: Recognize the findings of alcohol dependence and its appropriate therapy for a hospitalized patient.

365. Answer: E

Answer: Reassure and encourage cessation of alcohol.
This constellation of signs and symptoms in a young male patient is consistent with the diagnosis of cluster headache, and this diagnosis can be made based on analysis of the history and physical exam. Because this patient has no disturbing findings to indicate a central mass (papilledema, cranial nerve palsies, or sensorimotor impairment), he does not need imaging of his brain. Cluster headaches typically occur in daily spells for about a week or so every 6-12 months. The headaches may last up to 3 hours, are associated with conjunctival injection, excessive tearing and rhinorrhea, and often occur at night. Alcohol, stress, seasonal changes, and allergens seem to precipitate events in some patients. Once a cluster has begun, removing the alcohol stimulus makes ensuing attacks less severe. While cluster attacks do seem to be related to histamine release, antihistamines do not help the attacks or the symptoms. Sumatriptan, ergotamine, and metoclopramide are the mainstays of pharmaceutical treatment for attacks. Antibiotics are not indicated, because this is not a case of sinusitis (headaches would be constant, not relenting). Cryptococcal meningitis does occur in non-immunosuppressed individuals, but symptoms are not clustered, and conjunctival irritation with increased lacrimation is not a feature.

Board Testing Point: Recognize the symptoms of cluster headache and recommend appropriate management.

366. Answer: B

Answer: Temporal artery biopsy.
The most likely diagnosis is temporal arteritis, a granulomatous inflammation that affects the medium and large vessels in persons over 55 years of age. Associated physical symptoms include those mentioned in the history; jaw claudication is present in > 50% of affected individuals. Although an MRI may be ordered to narrow the differential, and the ESR is typically > 100, the biopsy will show multinucleated giant cells, the pathological hallmark of this illness. The other choices, including the ESR, are not going to be diagnostic because they are nonspecific.

Board Testing Point: Recognize that a temporal artery biopsy is the diagnostic test of choice for temporal arteritis.

367. Answer: B

Answer: Prednisone.
For temporal arteritis, prednisone is usually given at a dose of 1 mg/kg (no greater than 80 mg/day), but the range of doses is 0.5 mg to 2 mg/kg/day. The goal of treatment is to reduce the pain and prevent vision loss. Blindness can be transient (like amaurosis fugax) or permanent (if the granulomatous inflammation causes an occlusion of the ophthalmic artery). The response to treatment is usually 1-3 days. Treatment continues until the patient is consistently improved and may be required for longer than 1 year in some cases. None of the other choices are first line therapy for temporal arteritis.

Board Testing Point: Prescribe the appropriate treatment for temporal arteritis.

368. Answer: C

Answer: Normal pressure hydrocephalus (NPH).
The question highlights a person with a *gradually* worsening dementia, which eliminates CJD from the differential, since CJD has a rapid onset and course. Although Alzheimer's and multi-infarct dementia can cause

memory problems, the triad of gait abnormalities (magnetic gait), incontinence, and dementia is "classic" for NPH.

In this illness, lumbar puncture (LP) is diagnostic, and can also be therapeutic. Some people will experience an improvement in their mental status temporarily after removal of a large volume of cerebral spinal fluid (CSF). Usually, it is this test in combination with an MRI that strongly supports the clinical history, thereby making the diagnosis of NPH. Parkinson disease results in a shuffling gait.

Board Testing Point: Identify normal pressure hydrocephalus as a diagnosis based on history and physical examination.

369. Answer: D

Answer: Oxygen.
This patient has cluster headaches, characterized by severe, unilateral headaches that last up to a few hours. Cluster headaches are more common in men than women and may be associated with nasal stuffiness, rhinorrhea, excessive tearing, stabbing pain near the eye, and sometimes nausea and vomiting. Decongestants, which are commonly prescribed for "sinus" headaches, are not helpful in cluster headaches. NSAIDs, including indomethacin, can be tried for first-line therapy in milder headaches, including migraines, but they have not been shown to be effective as abortive therapy for cluster headaches. Amitriptyline may be helpful in chronic tension-type headaches and for prophylaxis of migraines. Prednisone has shown some utility as prophylaxis for cluster headaches, but this agent is not recommended because of its side effects. Inhaled oxygen therapy (6-15 L by nasal cannula for fifteen minutes) has been shown to give dramatic relief of cluster headaches and has essentially no side effects. Sumatriptan, especially in combination with nasal oxygen, is also effective.

Board Testing Point: Recognize the symptoms of cluster headache and prescribe urgent treatment.

370. Answer: C

Answer: Ferritin level.
This patient has symptoms consistent with restless legs syndrome (RLS). As many as 20-30% of patients with this syndrome may have low iron levels. Replacement of iron can relieve the restless legs symptoms. Usually, a cutoff of 50 is used for ferritin, treating those with iron if their ferritin levels are less than 50. Pharmacotherapy can be employed in patients with normal ferritin levels and RLS. Of the choices listed, only ferritin would be useful in diagnosis.

Board Testing Point: Identify critical information needed for the diagnosis of RLS.

371. Answer: C

Answer: Migraine headache.
Migraines are more common in women, but can also occur in young men as well. There are no focal neurological findings or papilledema, which eliminates both pseudotumor and CNS tumor from the differential. The description of this headache supports the diagnosis of migraine more so than cluster or tension headache or subarachnoid hemorrhage. The description of an aura (the flashing lights) suggests a "classic migraine."

Board Testing Point: Diagnose migraine headache.

372. Answer: A

Answer: Pseudotumor cerebri.
Idiopathic intracranial hypertension usually occurs in obese, premenopausal women. Obesity appears to have a strong causal association with pseudotumor cerebri. Some drugs also can cause it, including glucocorticoids, tetracycline, and vitamin A. Symptoms include headache and horizontal diplopia. There is almost always a peripheral visual field loss, which is commonly asymptomatic. Papilledema is the hallmark finding on exam. CT/MRI and CSF pressure > 250 mm H_2O confirm the diagnosis. Acetazolamide is helpful as is furosemide.

Board Testing Point: Recognize symptoms of pseudotumor cerebri in patients complaining of headache and peripheral visual field loss.

373. Answer: C

Answer: Restless leg syndrome (RLS).
RLS is manifested by spontaneous, continuous leg movements and paresthesias, often worse at rest and while sleeping. Patients often pace the floor to help relieve symptoms. Diagnosis is made based upon typical symptoms and a normal exam, including neurological exam, which this patient had. The normal exam also helps to rule out DVT, myositis, vascular disease, and spinal stenosis as the cause of the symptoms. Hypokalemia may cause muscular and neurologic symptoms, but the regularity and severity of this patient's features are very consistent with RLS. Stain-induced myopathy would produce muscle pain and weakness.

Board Testing Point: Recognize symptoms of restless leg syndrome.

374. Answer: B

Answer: Lumbar spinal stenosis.
Lumbar spinal stenosis is characterized by worsening symptoms with walking and standing, but improvement with sitting or squatting. Claudication will cause worse symptoms with walking but improvement with standing and sitting. A positive straight leg raising (Lasègue's sign) test is absent in lumbar stenosis but will produce pain in those patients with herniated lumbar discs with ipsilateral radicular pain secondary to nerve root compression. Patrick's sign (lateral rotation of the flexed knee) implies ipsilateral degenerative hip joint disease.

Board Testing Point: Recognize the findings of lumbar spinal stenosis and differentiate them from other causes of lower extremity pain.

375. Answer: B

Answer: A decreased ankle jerk reflex will be seen with S1 radiculopathy.
This is the physical finding that will help differentiate S1 radiculopathy from sciatica. Both conditions will result in the patient not being able to stand on his toes. Foot drop occurs with L5 radiculopathy or peroneal nerve injury, not with either of these conditions.

Board Testing Point: Be able to differentiate S1 radiculopathy from sciatica using ankle jerk reflexes as a discriminator.

376. Answer: A

Answer: He will be able to invert his foot with peroneal nerve injury, but will not be able to with L5 radiculopathy.
Peroneal nerve compression usually occurs at the proximal head of the fibula, causing foot drop. L5 radiculopathy also causes foot drop. To distinguish between the two: Patients with peroneal nerve compression cannot evert the foot well but can still invert it, while patients with L5 radiculopathy cannot evert or invert their foot. Also with L5 radiculopathy, the hamstrings and thigh abductors will be weak and are not affected by peroneal nerve compression. If you think of where the peroneal nerve compression occurs, this makes sense because anything "above" the compression will be fine.

Board Testing Point: Differentiate between peroneal nerve injury and L5 radiculopathy based on simple physical exam findings.

377. Answer: A

Answer: CT or MRI of the brain.
The differential of a left hemiparesis and coma includes CNS tumor, stroke, focal hemorrhage (possibly due to uncontrolled severe hypertension), and a lobar hemorrhage due to amyloid. Neuroimaging must be performed as soon as possible. CT is in most instances more readily available.

Although serum glucose and calcium labs are likely to be performed, neither would explain focal findings on the neurological exam. An LP would be potentially dangerous, since it may worsen the herniation and should not be performed without imaging first, given the focal exam findings. An EEG would not be an initial test in this setting since it would be unlikely to provide diagnostic information.

Board Testing Point: Recognize the need for intracranial imaging in the setting of upper motor neuron deficits with coma.

378. Answer: B

Answer: Pramipexole.
In patients with adequate iron stores, treatment with dopaminergic drugs is the most beneficial treatment for restless leg syndrome (RLS). Pramipexole is effective and has been well tolerated. Levodopa with carbidopa is another reasonable option. In resistant cases, low-dose benzodiazepines can be helpful. Antidepressants, oxycodone, and topiramate are not first-line therapies for RLS. Referral to a sleep specialist would be appropriate if she fails to respond to pramipexole.

Board Testing Point: Synthesize appropriate pharmaceutical treatment of restless leg syndrome (RLS).

379. Answer: C

Answer: Dropout of dopamine-producing cells in the substantia nigra of the midbrain.
He has all of the clinical signs and symptoms of Parkinson disease. Four major characteristics are seen: Resting tremor, Rigidity and flexed posture, Retarded movement, and loss of postural Reflexes (the 4 R's). Demyelination is seen with multiple sclerosis. Progressive supranuclear palsy causes a similar disease to Parkinson disease, but those affected do not have a tremor and tend to have erect posture with hyperextension of the neck. Arsenic toxicity would result in more global findings.

Board Testing Point: Recognize the clinical findings of Parkinson disease and the pathologic lesion responsible.

---

380. Answer: C

Answer: Vertical ophthalmoplegia.
Usually within 2 years of diagnosis, patients with progressive supranuclear palsy develop vertical ophthalmoplegia. This causes the patient to be unable to voluntarily look up or down, and eventually progresses to ophthalmoplegia in all directions of gaze. When this occurs, the patient has difficulty with reading, eating, and walking down stairs. Within another 2-3 years, patients may be unable to walk, primarily because of marked balance impairment. There is no specific treatment.

Board Testing Point: Know that progressive supranuclear palsy results in vertical and eventual total ophthalmoplegia.

---

381. Answer: C

Answer: Iron deficiency and renal failure can produce these symptoms.
This scenario is most consistent with restless leg syndrome (RLS), a disorder of dysesthesias of the legs and feet and less commonly the upper extremities. The symptoms are worsened with inactivity and often occur related to sleep time. Caffeine, fatigue and pregnancy also tend to worsen symptoms. Dopaminergic agents such as ropinirole are generally very effective at relieving symptoms and are the preferred treatment. RLS often includes periodic leg movements, although not all RLS patients experience the myoclonic limb complaints. Symptoms of claudication are worsened, not improved, with increased activity and although rest symptoms can occur, it is generally in the company of severe daytime complaints as well. Both iron deficiency and renal failure can lead to RLS symptoms, though in these circumstances this is a secondary and not a primary disease process.

Board Testing Point: Recognize the findings associated with restless leg syndrome.

---

382. Answer: A

Answer: Sumatriptan.
She has classic migraine headaches infrequently, and would benefit from an abortive agent, such as sumatriptan, as opposed to a prophylactic agent (valproate, propranolol, verapamil, and amitriptyline). While propranolol and amitriptyline are used for migraine prophylaxis, verapamil is perhaps more effective in cluster headache.

Board Testing Point: Manage the pharmaceutical treatment of migraine headache.

---

383. Answer: B

Answer: Parkinson disease.
Since he is on no medications, he does not have a drug-induced Parkinsonism (not a choice here). Shy-Drager by definition includes severe orthostasis. Striatonigral degeneration looks like Parkinson's without the resting tremor. PSP includes loss of voluntary vertical gaze and axial rigidity (more than appendicular). PSP is also highly associated with dementia. Alzheimer's and Parkinson's can overlap; however, Alzheimer's does not begin with these symptoms, and is therefore very unlikely.

Board Testing Point: Recognize the characteristics of Parkinson disease.

384. Answer: B

Answer: Tensilon test.
She has a characteristic presentation of myasthenia gravis. The age of onset is between the second and fourth decades of life. Myasthenia is due to circulating polyclonal IgG autoantibodies (produced by B-lymphocytes) to the acetylcholine receptor. It is characterized by weakness that worsens with physical activity. In about 40% of cases, the presenting complaint is diplopia. Other common symptoms include dysarthria, dysphagia, and decreased range of facial movements. Limb and neck weakness is common. It is uncommon for the limbs to be affected without other symptoms. Medications such as D-penicillamine (once used to treat rheumatoid arthritis) can cause drug-induced myasthenia. If the drug is discontinued, the myasthenia-like syndrome resolves. Although TIA and stroke must be considered in the diagnosis, it is very unusual for ischemia to produce diplopia alone. Often, other neurological symptoms are present. Graves ophthalmopathy must always be considered when a patient has diplopia. Often, physical signs of Graves disease, such as the Graves stare, will suggest a diagnosis of thyroid disease.

The first diagnostic test is the Tensilon test. When clinical signs are present (not just subjective diplopia), the Tensilon test can confirm the clinical diagnosis. Tensilon (edrophonium) is a short-acting acetylcholinesterase inhibitor that acts to prolong the effects of acetylcholine at the postsynaptic neuromuscular junction. This will reverse the weakness transiently. A positive test, then, would be improvement in clinical signs. A second test is the acetylcholine receptor antibody test. It is positive in 50% of patients with ocular myasthenia, and positive in 90% of patients with generalized myasthenia. In this case (ocular symptoms only), it would be a second-line test. CT of the chest would be indicated to eliminate the possibility of a thymoma, which is present in about 15% of patients with myasthenia gravis. EMG may be performed as a confirmatory test as well. The classic EMG finding in myasthenia gravis is the electro-decremental response to repetitive stimulation. An MRI of the brain would not be needed.

Board Testing Point: Recognize the characteristics of myasthenia gravis and describe how to diagnose it.

RHEUMATOLOGY

385. Answer: C

Answer: Felty syndrome.
The patient's steroid-requiring arthritis, the ulnar deviations and limited range of motion, and the inflammatory nature and location of involvement (small joints) all suggest rheumatoid arthritis. She has splenomegaly on exam and granulocytopenia, this combination in patients with rheumatoid arthritis (RA) is consistent with Felty syndrome. The diagnosis is made in patients whose neutrophil count is < 2000 cells/mm³ and who have splenomegaly, usually in association with severe RA. Evan syndrome is the combination of autoimmune hemolysis plus immune thrombocytopenia. Typically, low-dose steroids will not cause myelosuppression. Amyloidosis may cause splenomegaly, and may be associated with uncontrolled rheumatic disease; however, neutropenia is not seen in this disorder. Gaucher disease is a lysosomal storage disease that causes splenomegaly and may cause thrombocytopenia but is not associated with neutropenia.

Board Testing Point: Interpret laboratories and a physical examination and diagnose Felty syndrome.

386. Answer: A

Answer: Begin calcium 1.5 gm and vitamin D 800 U.
This patient has osteopenia but does not meet criteria for osteoporosis. She should receive calcium and vitamin D. Based on her T scores, the number needed to treat (NNT) to prevent one fracture is > 500 patients for bisphosphonates and probably higher for raloxifene. She does not meet current guidelines for preventative treatment.

Current guidelines suggest treatment for postmenopausal women with T-score < -2.5 in the absence of risk factors and < -2.0 in the presence of these risk factors:
- Personal history of fracture before age 40
- Family history of fracture in a first-degree relative
- Current cigarette smoking
- Body weight < 127 lbs., regardless of height.

The website www.osteoed.org has case-based learning available for practice.

Board Testing Point: Interpret T scores and prescribe therapy for osteopenia.

387. Answer: B

Answer: Cotton-wool appearance on skull films.
This is a case of Paget disease of bone. Paget's is often found on routine lab testing (elevated alkaline phosphatase), since it is usually asymptomatic. Calcium levels are usually normal. Paget lesions are metabolically active and would light up on bone scan, which tests for osteoblastic (not osteoclastic) activity; however, skull or long-bone films are likely to show the classic feature of Paget's: "osteitis deformans." Hearing loss may occur from bony involvement of the skull. In patients with widely metastatic prostate cancer, bone scan would show increased osteoblastic activity, but a higher PSA might be expected, and SPEP would not show a monoclonal spike. Patients with hyperparathyroidism and malignancy-related PTHrP elevations should have elevated serum calcium levels. Patients with multiple myeloma may have hypercalcemia and an abnormal SPEP, but myeloma rarely lights up on bone scan (myeloma is primarily an osteoclastic bone disease).

Board Testing Point: Interpret laboratory tests, diagnose Paget disease of bone and characterize abnormalities seen in Paget disease.

388. Answer: D

Answer: IV cefotaxime and vancomycin.
In febrile patients with known RA and an unusual or acute flare of joint pain, you must suspect septic arthritis. Joint aspirate should be performed. Antibiotic therapy is warranted if the joint fluid is purulent, has a positive Gram stain, the WBC count is markedly elevated (> 50,000-100,000), or the joint fluid is inflammatory (elevated WBC count) with no other explanation. Oral or IM glucocorticoids or NSAIDs (e.g., ketorolac) will obviously not be effective in septic arthritis. Intraarticular glucocorticoids may lead to joint erosion/destruction in patients with bacterial arthritis. *Staph aureus* and *Streptococcus* are common causes of bacterial arthritis, but there is an increased incidence of Gram-negative infections in patients who are immunosuppressed; thus, empiric treatment with coverage for both Gram-positive and Gram-negative organisms is warranted in this patient.

Board Testing Point: Recognize septic arthritis in a patient with underlying joint disease.

389. Answer: C

Answer: Enalapril 1.25 mg IV q 6 hours; first dose now.
This is a case of scleroderma renal crisis with malignant hypertension. In diffuse scleroderma, renal crisis is one of the most serious early complications. This is usually seen in young women with early rapid progression of this disease. African-American patients with diffuse disease have a much higher incidence of renal crisis compared to Caucasian counterparts (21% compared to 7%). Differential diagnosis for this presentation in a patient without obvious scleroderma would include HUS, TTP, antiphospholipid antibody syndrome and malignant nephrosclerosis in those with pre-existing hypertension. But in settings where scleroderma is a known diagnosis, the diagnosis is straightforward. Screening for this complication in diffuse scleroderma patients is helpful in preventing renal failure; blood pressure should be monitored monthly and renal function monitored q 3 months. ACE inhibitors can prevent this complication and treat renal crisis, even in the setting of acute renal failure. ACE-I also appear to reduce mortality. This complication was seen in up to 25% of patients in the past but much less often now due to the use of ACE inhibitors. Calcium channel blockers are typically added when ACE-I fail to control the blood pressure adequately. Beta-blockers and diuretics are not known to exert any affect on reversing the renal disease in these patients. Isosorbide and hydralazine in combination are used to treat African-American patients with heart failure, not for scleroderma renal crisis.

Malignant hypertension, plus acute renal failure, microangiopathic hemolytic anemia, and retinal hemorrhages would be the expected findings with scleroderma. Again, ACE inhibitors, not beta-blockers, are the drugs of choice to prevent and treat renal crisis.

Board Testing Point: Diagnose scleroderma renal crisis and prescribe Ace-Inhibitors for treatment.

390. Answer: C

Answer: Joint deformities.
Localized scleroderma causes either morphea, patches of skin thickening, or linear scleroderma, long limb-length areas of skin thickening that may overlay the joints. Linear scleroderma can overlay joints, causing contractures and deformities. Localized disease does not lead to diffuse disease ("systemic sclerosis"), systemic vascular effects (such as renal crisis and Raynaud phenomenon) and pulmonary hypertension. Localized scleroderma is much more common in children than adults. Morphea is usually much less clinically significant than linear

scleroderma. Linear scleroderma through the face is termed "en coup de sabre," and this can be quite disfiguring. Still, localized scleroderma is not a systemic disease.

Board Testing Point: Identify differences between localized scleroderma and diffuse systemic sclerosis.

391. Answer: B

Answer: Immune complexes around muscle fibrils.
This patient has dermatomyositis. Muscle biopsy in a patient with dermatomyositis will show infiltration of muscle fibers with lymphocytes that is more intense around vessels. Immunohistochemical analysis will reveal immune complex deposition in the areas of inflammatory infiltrate. EMG will show primarily myopathic changes. PFTs in patients whose lungs are affected may show restrictive changes with decreased volumes and low DLCO. Ordering cancer screening studies is inappropriate in this patient since, overall, only about 15% of adults with dermatomyositis have a malignancy, and she is only 25 years old. However, the number of patients with cancer increases to ~ 30% in adults over 65 years of age. Urine is usually normal in dermatomyositis. Complete blood count and ESR are also usually normal; CK, aldolase, LDH, ALT, and/or AST are elevated in most patients.

Inflammatory myositis causes proximal muscle weakness and, in dermatomyositis, the classic rash (heliotrope and Gottron papules) is virtually pathognomonic for this diagnosis. Malignancy association is not present in children or usually in young adults, but the risk increases with age. The investigation of inflammatory myositis may involve a series of laboratory and diagnostic testing including muscle biopsy, EMG, and sometimes MRI of muscles showing edema of proximal muscle groups.

Board Testing Point: Predict the pathology in the muscles in dermatomyositis.

392. Answer: A

Answer: Slippage of the L5 vertebra relative to the body of the S1 vertebra.

This patient has spondylolysis, a defect in the pars interarticularis. Repetitive flexion exercises during activities such as gymnastics, wrestling or ballet dancing often results in this injury. Slippage of the affected vertebrae, termed spondylolisthesis, is the most common complication. Acute urinary retention is a possible but uncommon complication. Patients with spondylolisthesis often have evidence of a sacral kyphosis, flattened buttocks and a prominent anterior abdominal wall.

Board Testing Point: Recognize spondylolysis and that the most common complication is spondylolisthesis.

393. Answer: B

Answer: Digital tuft resorption.
In severe scleroderma changes, ulcerations form on the tips of the fingers with occasional osteomyelitis that gradually results in loss of the tips of the fingers. The severe skin thickening and tightness causes contractures of the digits as well. Note the telangiectasias over the palms. These changes are typical for severe CREST or limited scleroderma but could also be found in diffuse scleroderma patients.

Digital tuft resorption is caused by progressive vascular changes associated with severe Raynaud's. Cutaneous vasculitis is not seen in the case of scleroderma, although one can see loss of the tips of the fingers in severe polyarteritis nodosa or rheumatoid vasculitis. With inflammatory polyarthritis, no loss of the fingertips would be seen due to arthritis, although finger contractures might be seen. Interosseous muscle weakness is not seen. The muscle weakness due to rheumatoid arthritis, for example, causes atrophy most obvious on the dorsum of the hands. Peripheral neuropathy causes weakness, atrophy, and contractures but no loss of fingertips.

Board Testing Point: Characterize the pathophysiology of scleroderma.

394. Answer: C

Answer: Azathioprine.
Allopurinol slows the metabolism of azathioprine and so must be dosed very carefully to avoid significant bone marrow suppression. Metoprolol, prednisone, and aspirin do not interact with allopurinol. If colchicine is used to treat the gout, renal failure may become an issue since cyclosporine increases the risk of toxicity from colchicine.

Board Testing Point: Recognize that gout is very common in heart transplant patients and that allopurinol-azathioprine interactions are a concern.

395. Answer: D

Answer: Loss of lumbar flexion.
Patients with ankylosing spondylitis (AS) first develop stiffness and loss of lumbar motion. The Schober test quantifies lumbar flexion and shows a decrease in these patients. Kyphotic thoracic deformity may develop as the disease progresses. Chest expansion decreases, not increases, in these patients as they develop thoracic involvement. Leg length discrepancy would be expected in the setting of hip or other lower extremity arthritis and are not described in this patient. Cervical fixation in flexion is one of the dreaded late complications as the spine fuses.

The physical findings of early AS involve loss of motion of the lumbar spine with caudal spread of the disease in most patients. Loss of extension of the thoracic and cervical spine and progressive fusion in a flexed position are later features. Current medications, plus appropriate physical therapy techniques, should minimize these complications.

Board Testing Point: Recognize the findings of ankylosing spondylitis.

396. Answer: D

Answer: Anterior uveitis.
Ankylosing spondylitis (AS) is one of the rheumatic diseases to occur more often in young men. Insidious onset of low back pain with > 1 hour of morning stiffness would be the typical presentation. Extraarticular complications are seen more often in those with +HLA B 27 (85-90%).

Anterior uveitis occurs in 25% of ankylosing spondylitis (AS) patients and may precede the joint symptoms. While aortitis, amyloidosis, apical pulmonary fibrosis, and cauda equina syndrome may occur in AS patients, they are much less common complications. Aortitis is uncommon and is found in ~ 5% of patients. Amyloidosis apical pulmonary fibrosis is rare, occurring in < 1% of cases. Apical pulmonary fibrosis is pathognomic of AS but is much less common than anterior uveitis. Cauda equina syndrome is also uncommon, occurring in < 5% of AS patients.

Board Testing Point: Recognize anterior uveitis as a common complication of ankylosing spondylitis.

397. Answer: A

Answer: Diffuse proliferative glomerulonephritis (DP-GN).
DP-GN is the form of glomerulonephritis with the greatest risk of progression to renal failure. About 50% of SLE patients develop some form of glomerulonephritis. DP-GN often presents with hypertension, hematuria, proteinuria, and sometimes with acute renal failure. A renal biopsy will diagnose DP-GN and establish chronicity giving prognostic information about the risk of renal failure.

FP-GN and mesangial GN are not as severe and may respond to a less potent treatment regimen. Interstitial nephritis is often seen as part of the pathologic picture of lupus nephritis, but it does not usually progress to renal failure. Membranous GN causes more severe nephrotic syndrome but is less likely to progress than DP-GN.

Board Testing Point: Recognize that diffuse proliferative glomerulonephritis is associated with progression to renal failure.

398. Answer: C

Answer: Osteoarthritis.
The radiograph reveals unilateral compartment narrowing laterally, as well as osteophyte formation. Diabetes can cause frozen shoulders, carpal tunnel syndrome, "diabetic stiff hand syndrome," and Charcot joints, but not the degenerative changes seen on this x-ray. Obesity is a risk factor for development of OA, but a patient who is 15 pounds overweight is not at increased risk (30% over ideal body weight increases the risk of OA of the knees 2-3 fold). Osteoporosis can occur in patients with RA, but radiographs in osteoporosis would show significant osteopenia, not osteophytes and asymmetric joint space narrowing. The knee x-ray would show symmetric joint space narrowing if RA was the main cause of the knee pain in this patient.

Patients can have both RA and OA. In addition, secondary OA develops following long-standing RA in many patients. The radiographic changes seen can help differentiate these diagnoses. In OA, one sees osteophytes and asymmetric joint changes, with greater effects on the weight-bearing areas of large joints. In RA, one sees osteopenia, erosions, and symmetric narrowing.

Board Testing Point: Diagnose osteoarthritis based on history and radiographs.

399. Answer: E

Answer: Polyarteritis nodosa (PAN).
This is a case of vasculitis. Systemic vasculitides should always be suspected in patients who appear ill and have no obvious etiology. Search for a focus of abnormality begins with screening blood work; in this case, abnormalities include hypoalbuminemia (suggesting a systemic disease), slight transaminase elevation (explained by the positive test for Hepatitis B surface antigen and core IgG, indicating this patient is a chronic carrier of HBV), and an active urine sediment. Knowing HBV does not cause systemic disease, you should consider systemic diseases, such as vasculitides, that are associated with HBV. Polyarteritis nodosa is well-known to associate with HBV. PAN is a systemic necrotizing vasculitis that typically affects the small and medium-sized muscular arteries. It affects multiple organ systems and is usually ANCA-negative. PAN affects men more than women (1.5:1 ratio). Microscopic polyangiitis may be P-ANCA-positive (also known as MPO-ANCA), as can Goodpasture's; Wegener's is C-ANCA-positive (PR3-ANCA). These ANCA-positive vasculitides cause pulmonary-renal syndromes, meaning they typically affect only the lungs and the kidneys. Lupus may present in a similar fashion (rash, renal disease), but ANA should be positive, and SLE is more commonly seen in women.

IgA nephropathy occurs when IgA deposits accumulate in the renal mesangium and the mesangium proliferates in a pathological way. IgA nephropathy is not associated with vascular inflammation.

Board Testing Point: Associate polyarteritis nodosa with chronic hepatitis B infection.

400. Answer: C

Answer: Heberden node.
Heberden nodes are due to osteophyte formation of the DIP joints. Bouchard nodes are the name given to osteophytes of the PIP joints. A ganglion cyst is a soft tissue bulge due to a synovial cyst that can form at any joint but is most often seen in wrists and knees. Occasionally, these cysts can occur over the DIP and PIP joints, but would be soft and fluid-filled, not bony as are Heberden nodes. Soft, somewhat rubbery, mobile rheumatoid nodules can develop in seropositive RA patients. These can appear over DIP joints but are not hard and bony. Tophi are a result of gout. These are soft, yellowish nodules that overlay joints and digits.

Physical findings of OA include evidence of osteophytes, such as the Heberden and Bouchard nodes. There is also squaring of the base of the thumb and crepitus of joints, especially the knees. These findings, along with a history of brief morning stiffness in the presence of normal inflammatory markers, confirm the diagnosis of OA.

Board Testing Point: Diagnose Heberden nodes.

401. Answer: E

Answer: An x-ray of the knees.
Plain films are most useful to diagnose OA, although the symptoms may precede radiographic changes by several years. Standing view of weight-bearing joints is the best technique to assess OA. ANA and RF have no diagnostic or predictive value in patients with OA. An MRI might be indicated subsequently to assess for mechanical derangement such as a torn meniscus, but is not as appropriate to make an initial diagnosis of OA. Sedimentation rate would be useful to assess a possible inflammatory arthritis, but the test will be normal in OA and is a non-specific study.

The physical exam findings are most important in making a diagnosis of OA. Plain radiographs, particularly standing films of the knees, are helpful to confirm the diagnosis and determine the severity of joint changes. The laboratory tests are more useful to rule out other diagnoses than to make a diagnosis of OA.

Board Testing Point: Evaluate a patient with possible osteoarthritis.

402. Answer: E

Answer: Hyaluronate.
The management of OA includes analgesia with acetaminophen and non-steroidal anti-inflammatory agents. Exercise and weight loss are also important aspects of treatment. Hyaluronate is a form of viscosupplementation. Intraarticular injections of this product, which is similar to glycosaminoglycan (a major component of synovial fluid), have been shown to help the symptoms of OA. Alendronate is a bisphosphonate indicated for osteoporosis, not osteoarthritis. Bromelain is a nutraceutical from the pineapple plant with purported, yet unproven, benefit for arthritis symptoms. Methotrexate is indicated for rheumatoid arthritis, but does not help the symptoms of OA. Tetracyclines are under investigation for use in managing OA, but currently have not been shown to help OA symptoms.

Board Testing Point: Viscosupplementation (hyaluronate) has been shown to help the symptoms of OA of the knees and is under investigation for use in shoulder and hip OA.

403. Answer: D

Answer: Acute pulmonary embolism.
Total joint replacement is a common orthopedic procedure, and it has changed the outlook for people with severe OA, especially of the knees and hips. The first days to weeks following surgery is the time of greatest risk for pulmonary emboli. Joint replacements have been the biggest advancement in the management of OA over the past few decades, but the biologic therapies are the most important change in the treatment of RA. Most patients are over 60 years of age at the time of surgery. Since the joint replacements last 10-20 years, surgeons prefer not to perform these procedures on younger patients. Loosening of the prosthesis may occur in ~ 5% of patients but is usually a late complication. The indications for joint replacement are joint pain and dysfunction. Deformity is not a primary indication for this procedure.

The key to this case is to calculate the A-a gradient and establish that a diffusion defect is present. Interpretation of the blood gas leads one to conclude that a respiratory alkalosis is present; and if considering the differential diagnosis of respiratory alkalosis, one might consider uncontrolled pain or delirium as a cause of this presentation. However, her medical history is not consistent with enough alcohol intake to cause withdrawal, and the respiratory alkalosis associated with pain is not associated with an elevated A-a gradient. The gradient for this patient is calculated as 19.73, with a normal gradient for her age = 14.25.

Board Testing Point: Recognize that pulmonary embolism is a complication of total joint replacement surgery; interpret a blood gas and calculate the A-a gradient to recognize a diffusion defect.

404. Answer: B

Answer: Gout.
Rheumatic and autoimmune diseases are diagnosed much more often in women than in men. The etiology of this gender difference is not totally clear, although estrogen has immunogenic effects and may play a role. Dermatomyositis and rheumatoid arthritis are 3-4x more common in females. JIA is 4-5x more common in girls. Osteoarthritis is diagnosed 2-3x more often in women than in men. However, gout is seen more often in males than females.

Board Testing Point: Recognize that most rheumatic diseases are more commonly seen in women compared to men, except for gout. An important clue to an etiology of an arthritis on the Boards!

405. Answer: C

Answer: Hemochromatosis.
Calcium pyrophosphate dihydrate (CPPD) crystals cause pseudogout. Although these crystals develop commonly in older patients with osteoarthritis, younger patients with metabolic disorders and endocrinopathies are also at risk for developing CPPD. Positively birefringent CPPD crystals can be found in patients with hemochromatosis. Patients with hyperparathyroidism and acromegaly also develop pseudogout. Alcohol abuse is associated with MSU crystals or gout, which are negatively birefringent crystals. Patients with heart transplants are at increased risk to develop gout but not pseudogout. Synovial fluid crystals typically are not seen in RA or Reiter syndrome patients.

sr suuz d. sd

Board Testing Point: Recognize that positively birefringent crystals are CPPD crystals and associated with pseudogout and that pseudogout is common in hemochromatosis.

406. Answer: E

Answer: Pseudogout (calcium pyrophosphate deposition).
The radiographic change of pseudogout is chondrocalcinosis, as noted on the x-ray. This is due to CPPD deposition in the cartilage. With degenerative arthritis or OA changes, one would expect to see osteophytes and asymmetric joint space narrowing. There is no evidence of a fracture. Gout shows no radiographic changes, unless there are tophaceous erosions, usually at the periphery of small joints.

CPPD can present with acute arthritis but can also be asymptomatic with chondrocalcinosis discovered serendipitously on x-ray, as in this case. CPPD can occur in patients with OA and can cause a destructive Charcot-like arthropathy.

Board Testing Point: Diagnose CPPD based on chondrocalcinosis visible in a radiograph.

407. Answer: A

Answer: Aplastic anemia.
Colchicine works well for acute crystal arthropathy if used promptly in the first 2-3 days of an exacerbation. This drug has potentially serious side effects and must be used with caution, especially in patients with creatinine > 2.0 mg/dl. Two forms are available: oral and intravenous. The IV formulation is associated with worse side effects than the oral, and the IV form should be used with extreme caution and only in situations where the provider has experience with IV colchicine.

Severe bone marrow toxicity can occur with colchicine. Patients with renal insufficiency are at particular risk for these bone marrow side effects, as well as at risk for neurotoxicity. Hepatic necrosis, acute renal failure, and exfoliative dermatitis are not expected side effects of colchicine. Diarrhea is a common side effect of colchicine and, if severe, it might be possible for hypovolemia to develop. Usually, the diarrhea is self-limited once the colchicine is discontinued, so shock would not be seen.

Board Testing Point: Predict side effects of colchicine.

408. Answer: B

Answer: Pain at the insertion of the Achilles tendon.
This is a case of psoriatic arthritis presenting as a spondyloarthropathy (clue = sacroiliac pain). In the spondyloarthropathies, inflammation at the entheses, followed by erosion, and then calcification is the hallmark of these disorders. The characteristic "bamboo spine" is caused by these changes.

The entheses are the insertion sites at which tendons and ligaments attach to bone. The spondyloarthropathies have a tendency to localize to the sacroiliac joints and lower extremity joints. There is a strong association with HLA B27, not HLA DR4, in these disorders. The ophthalmologic complication most often associated with these disorders is acute anterior uveitis, not keratoconjunctivitis sicca. Delayed reflexes are observed in hypothyroidism.

Board Testing Point: Forecast that spondyloarthropathies affect the entheses.

409. Answer: D

Answer: Native American.
Up to 15% of some Native American populations may be affected by ankylosing spondylitis (AS). The second most commonly affected group is Caucasians of Northern European descent, with prevalence of 0.5-1.0%. AS is uncommon in African-American, Asian, and Hispanic populations.

AS has a strong genetic association with HLA B27. Up to 90% of people diagnosed with AS carry this genetic haplotype. In Caucasians, 7-8% of unaffected individuals are HLA B27+, whereas the occurrence of this haplotype is much higher in some Native Americans, up to 13%.

Board Testing Points: Identify ethnic groups that have a high association with ankylosing spondylitis. Remember for the Boards they won't give you someone's ethnicity unless it is clinically important!

410. Answer: D

Answer: X-ray of the sacroiliac joints.
Apical pulmonary fibrosis is a rare, but pathognomic, complication of ankylosing spondylitis (AS). Diffuse interstitial fibrosis is a more usual pulmonary manifestation of other autoimmune diseases, such as SLE, dermatomyositis and RA. A CT scan of the chest would not confirm the diagnosis of AS but would further define the apical fibrosis.

Sometimes, the extraarticular features of autoimmune diseases can suggest and confirm the diagnosis, as in this case. In AS, anterior uveitis is common (25%) and mandates yearly eye examinations. Cardiac manifestations, including aortic root dilation and arrhythmias, occur in ~ 5% and are among the most serious complications of this disease.

Board Testing Point: Recognize that pulmonary fibrosis is a pathognomic complication of ankylosing spondylitis.

411. Answer: B

Answer: Psoriatic arthritis.
Dactylitis is also seen in Reiter syndrome (also called seronegative spondyloarthropathy or reactive arthritis). Dactylitis is due to a combination of synovitis, enthesitis, and tenosynovitis. This causes diffuse inflammation of the digit, giving an appearance similar to a sausage.

Small joint involvement is not typical in ankylosing spondylitis (AS). Although small joint polyarthritis is characteristic of RA and SLE, dactylitis is not usually part of the scenario. In osteoarthritis, small joint involvement is common, but you would not see "sausage digits."

Board Testing Point: Recognize the findings associated with psoriatic arthritis.

412. Answer: B

Answer: Eyes.
This is a straightforward case of Reiter syndrome, a known association of urethritis, arthritis (especially including involvement of entheses, such as the Achilles tendons) and conjunctivitis. Urethritis is the first symptom,

followed by conjunctivitis and then arthritis. Arthritis is never the initial manifestation. Mucositis is a common feature and occurs about the same time as the conjunctivitis. Arthritis is a requisite for Reiter's (also called seronegative spondyloarthropathy or reactive arthritis).

Reiter syndrome causes urethritis regardless of the site of the triggering infections, GI, or GU origin. Following urethritis, conjunctivitis and mucositis occur, followed quickly by spondyloarthritis. Large joint asymmetric arthritis, tenosynovitis, enthesitis, and dactylitis are the typical joint manifestations.

Board Testing Point: Recognize the findings associated with Reiter's (also called seronegative spondyloarthropathy or reactive arthritis).

413. Answer: C

Answer: Infection.
Over the past 30 years, disability in patients with RA has dropped over 40% due to aggressive treatment. This is due to the use of methotrexate and, more recently, biologic agents such as etanercept. Infections are the most concerning potential side effects of the new class of biologic therapies. Bone marrow effects with red cell aplasia and increases in liver function tests have been rarely reported with the use of etanercept. Hypercoagulability is not a side effect of etanercept; nor is alopecia, although alopecia does occur with leflunomide.

Infections, especially tuberculosis and opportunistic organisms, are increased with the use of these newer agents. Careful monitoring and treatment of potential infections are critical for optimal management of these patients. Prescreening with the purified protein derivative (PPD) is used to assess risks for development of tuberculosis on treatment.

Board Testing Point: Identify potential side effects of etanercept.

414. Answer: C

Answer: WBC < 2000 cells/mm^3 with < 25% PMNs, glucose equal to serum, T. protein 1-3 g/dL, yellow in color and translucent.
Interpretation of joint aspiration is necessary both for the Boards and for clinical practice. We have presented 4 different situations in our answer selections. Option A represents "inflammatory" joint fluid, often characteristic of inflammatory but not infectious etiologies, such as rheumatoid arthritis, gout and, sometimes, trauma. Option B represents "septic" joint fluid; notice the very low glucose and the significant leukocytosis. Option C represents "noninflammatory" joint fluid, consistent with a diagnosis of osteoarthritis. Option D represents "hemorrhagic" joint fluid consistent with a diagnosis of hemarthrosis.

Board Testing Point: Differentiate etiologies of arthritis based on synovial fluid studies.

415. Answer: E

Answer: Calcium and vitamin D.
This patient does not need to be on bisphosphonate, raloxifene, or teriparatide. T scores reflect the amount of bone present relative to that of a young adult of the same gender with peak bone mass. A score > -1 is considered normal. Osteopenia is defined as T scores between -1 and -2.5. Osteoporosis is defined as T scores below -2.5. Her T scores are not low enough to recommend these therapies (recommended with T scores below -2.5). Calcium and vitamin D supplementation would be appropriate.

Board Testing Point: Interpret DEXA scan T scores and prescribe treatment for osteoporosis.

416. Answer: A

Answer: Testicular biopsy for confirmation of diagnosis.
This is a case of polyarteritis nodosa (PAN). Testicular biopsy identifies organ-specific involvement. Screening for hepatitis B is appropriate since a minority of cases of PAN is associated with chronic hepatitis B infection. But hepatitis A infection has not been shown to be associated with PAN. The initial use of plasmapheresis is not an established first-line treatment for polyarteritis nodosa.

Board Testing Point: Refer a patient with suspected PAN testicular involvement for biopsy to confirm polyarteritis nodosa.

417. Answer: B

Answer: Avascular necrosis.
This patient likely suffers from avascular necrosis (AVN), or osteonecrosis. > 90% of patients diagnosed with osteonecrosis either 1) use alcohol excessively or 2) use chronic steroids for underlying disease. 9% of patients with AVN have one of the following diagnoses: sickle cell anemia, Caisson disease, Gaucher disease, renal failure, chronic pancreatitis or HIV. The pathogenesis of the disease is not known, but men outnumber women with the condition 8 to 1. Average age at diagnosis is usually < 40 years. AVN presents insidiously as pain, initially with weight bearing, then later at rest. AVN specifically of the hip presents as groin or buttock pain. Any patient with the risk factor of chronic alcohol use who complains of pain in the groin and/or buttock should be evaluated for AVN.

Hungry bone syndrome is associated with hyperparathyroidism and does not cause pain. Hyperparathyroidism can cause bone pain, but he does not have any of the other symptoms of hyperparathyroidism, and given his alcohol use, he is at greater risk for AVN. B-12 deficiency does not cause groin pain. Paget disease is a disorder marked by increased bone resorption, but most patients are asymptomatic.

Board Testing Point: Diagnose avascular necrosis based on risk factors and physical examination.

418. Answer: C

Answer: Amyloidosis of the kidney.
In several inflammatory conditions (RA, ankylosing spondylitis, chronic infections, neoplasms), deposition of serum amyloid A protein (SAA) can occur if inflammation is not controlled. The kidney is the most commonly affected organ when deposition of SAA occurs. Nephrotic syndrome is the most common presentation, but other manifestations can occur when the protein deposits in vascular or tubular parts of the kidney (renal failure, nephrogenic diabetes insipidus). Fusion of SI joints occurs in long-standing untreated ankylosing spondylitis, not RA. Avascular necrosis and cataract formation occur as a result of long-term steroid use. Reactivation tuberculosis can occur in the setting of RA treated with anti-TNF agents, but this is not seen in patients with uncontrolled or untreated RA.

Board Testing Point: Predict secondary amyloidosis as a complication of poorly managed rheumatoid arthritis.

419. Answer: C

Answer: Diffuse fibrin thrombi and areas of fibrinoid necrosis.
This is a case of scleroderma renal crisis with malignant hypertension. In diffuse scleroderma, renal crisis is one of the most serious early complications. This is usually seen in young women with early rapid progression of this disease. African-American patients with diffuse disease have a much higher incidence of renal crisis compared to Caucasian counterparts (21% compared to 7%). Differential diagnosis for this presentation in a patient without obvious scleroderma would include HUS, TTP, antiphospholipid antibody syndrome, and malignant nephrosclerosis in those with pre-existing hypertension. But in settings where scleroderma is a known diagnosis, the diagnosis is straightforward, and renal biopsy is not indicated.

Were a renal biopsy to be performed, pathology would reveal fibrin thrombi and areas of fibrinoid necrosis. Diffuse scleroderma causes proliferation of normal connective tissue with vascular disease due to vascular wall thickening and narrowing of the lumen. Hence, renal disease in diffuse scleroderma is akin to bilateral renal artery stenosis. The stenotic lumen comes about through a series of pathologic changes, and what you see in a renal biopsy is determined by the time period in which you sample the kidney. This is the described sequence of events:

Fibrin thrombi and areas of fibrinoid necrosis seen in the arcuate and interlobular arteries and glomeruli → healing of these areas with mucoid intimal thickening → concentric "onion-skin" hypertrophy of interlobular arteries. So the mucoid intimal thickening and "onion-skin" will occur much later in the process after this acute attack, which has diffuse fibrin thrombi and fibrinoid necrosis.

Crescentic glomerulonephritis and immune complex depositions are pathology types seen in etiologies of glomerulonephritis, a condition characterized by active urine sediment and not present in this clinical scenario. Only three disorders present with linear IgG staining in glomeruli visible by IF: diabetic nephropathy, fibrillary glomerulonephritis, and anti-GBM antibody disease (Goodpasture's).

Board Testing Point: Predict the renal pathology in scleroderma renal crisis.

420. Answer: C

Answer: Counsel her that transient thrombocytopenia and leukopenia may be seen in her children.
ANA-negative lupus clearly carries risk to the fetus in the setting of a positive SSA antibody, which increases the risk of 3rd degree heart block. So this patient and her child are at risk for untoward effects from her SLE, and she should not be counseled otherwise. Neonatal lupus transmission can present as heart block, cardiomyopathy, rash of the skin, or abnormalities such as transient thrombocytopenia or leukopenia. Pre-existing lupus nephritis can be flared by pregnancy, but nephritis is not increased in patients with SLE who become pregnant but do not have pre-existing renal disease. Hydroxychloroquine and prednisone can be continued through pregnancy if necessary.

Board Testing Point: Counsel patients appropriately on the risks of SLE with SSA antibodies and pregnancy.

421. Answer: C

Answer: After treating his acute attack, consider switching his antihypertensive treatment from HCTZ to a different antihypertensive.
Hydrochlorothiazide is known to cause retention of uric acid by stimulating a net increase in reabsorption of urate at the proximal tubule of the kidney. Given that the first attack of gout has occurred within six months of institution of hydrochlorothiazide, discontinuation of this medication is appropriate if an alternative treatment for hypertension can be instituted. The diagnosis of gout can be confirmed only by demonstrating the presence of

intracellular negatively birefringent uric acid crystals on joint fluid analysis. The serum uric acid does not confirm this diagnosis. With diagnosis, appropriate treatment does include use of NSAIDs. Allopurinol, however, should never be instituted or discontinued in the setting of an acute gouty attack. Hypothyroidism, hemochromatosis, and hyperparathyroidism are three causes of calcium pyrophosphate crystal disease (CPPD or "pseudogout"). Pseudogout is associated with positively birefringent, rhomboid-shaped crystals in synovial fluid. The negatively birefringent crystals in his fluid establish his diagnosis definitively as gout (monosodium urate crystal deposition disease). Checking for TSH, ferritin, and calcium is not indicated with this clinical picture.

Board Testing Point: Interpret history and joint fluid studies to diagnose gout; recommend discontinuation of a thiazide diuretic in a new diagnosis of gout.

422. Answer: D

Answer: Prescribe allopurinol with close follow-up of coagulation studies.
This question tests your knowledge of drug interactions with allopurinol, a frequently prescribed drug in middle-age patients who present with hyperuricemia and gout. In most patients, allopurinol raises warfarin levels and can result in prolonged coagulation studies and bleeding. PT and PTT tests should be monitored aggressively after the prescription of allopurinol to a patient taking warfarin. Allopurinol also raises theophylline levels and increases the risk of marrow suppression when combined with azathioprine, 6-mercaptopurine and cyclophosphamide. COX-2 inhibitors should not be prescribed to patients with a history of coronary artery disease if alternative treatments are available. In this patient, future flares should be managed with intra-articular injections followed by oral colchicine for refractory cases only since this patient is at greater risk for colchicine-induced renal failure given his comorbidities.

Board Testing Point: Characterize allopurinol drug interactions.

423. Answer: D

Answer: Anti-Sm antibodies are seen in approximately 25% of patients with SLE.
Anti-Sm (anti-Smith) antibodies are seen in approximately 25% of patients with systemic lupus erythematosus. While the sensitivity of this test is low at 25%, this is a highly specific test and is seen only in SLE. Anti-sclerotic 70 is associated with diffuse systemic sclerosis (scleroderma). Anti-centromere antibody is associated with limited systemic sclerosis or CREST. Anti-histone antibodies are associated with drug-induced lupus. Drug-induced lupus classically does not cause renal or central nervous system disease. Finally, RNP antibodies are associated with mixed connective tissue disease. The rare association of heart block in children born to patients with lupus is associated with SSA/SSB antibody.

Board Testing Point: Interpret serology used in the diagnosis of connective tissue diseases.

424. Answer: D

Answer: White blood cells on urinalysis.
She most likely has reactive arthritis or Reiter syndrome. Symptoms often follow an enteric (*Shigella*, *Salmonella*, or *Yersinia*) or venereal (*Chlamydia*) infection and include conjunctivitis or uveitis, arthritis, and dysuria mimicking a urinary tract infection. Although pyuria is common, urine cultures are negative, consistent with a nonbacterial urethritis. Reiter Syndrome is considered to be a seronegative (ANA and RF negative) spondyloarthropathy as is ankylosing spondylitis. Both may be associated with HLA-B27 although this finding is far more common in ankylosing spondylitis. Red cell casts would be seen with glomerulonephritis,

thrombocytopenia would not be associated with her findings, and elevated liver enzymes are unlikely as well. She has no findings either for a urinary tract infection, so culturing *E. coli* is not likely.

Board Testing Point: Recognize the findings of reactive arthritis (Reiter syndrome) in a patient with recent GI or GU infection.

ALLERGY / IMMUNOLOGY

425. Answer: C

Answer: Perform sputum washings to detect possible eosinophils or neutrophils.
Sputum washings demonstrating the presence of eosinophils or neutrophils is consistent with the diagnosis of occupational asthma. Certain professions increase the risk of airway disease arising from exposure to workplace irritants, including farmers, cotton workers, and individuals exposed to cedar dust. Bakeries are noted for the presence of multiple airway irritants such as cereal particles, molds, and egg proteins. Eosinophils and/or neutrophils are present in the sputum of most individuals with an established diagnosis of occupational asthma. Many airway complaints arise from inflammation and chronic swelling of the respiratory tract and may not demonstrate a clinically significant response to inhaled bronchodilators. Skin testing can be helpful in identifying potential offending agents but testing reagent is not available for all workplace substances. In addition, a positive skin test result only documents exposure and sensitization to a potential allergen, but does not prove a causative effect with airway symptoms. The diagnosis of occupational asthma is based on clinical judgment and benefits from serial airflow measurements, both at work and during periods away from the workplace. Unless the symptoms are life-threatening, removal from work can impede the diagnostic process and can also impose significant financial hardship.

Board Testing Point: Recommend the correct test for diagnosis of occupational asthma.

426. Answer: B

Answer: Oral decongestants.
Vasomotor rhinitis produces clear nasal discharge secondary to congestion of the nasal mucosa. Alternating exposure to dry and humid or to cold and warm environments can trigger this problem. Review of this scenario reveals no evidence of an infectious or allergic cause for this patient's drainage. Steroids, antibiotics, and anti-histamines are not primary treatments for vasomotor rhinitis. Nasal alpha-agonists run the risk of inducing rebound nasal congestion, rhinitis medicamentosa. Oral decongestants and modification of environmental exposures are the most appropriate interventions.

Board Testing Point: Diagnose and treat vasomotor rhinitis.

427. Answer: A

Answer: Nickel sensitivity.
Linear rashes most commonly reflect an external source for the rash. The distribution of the rash in this scenario is consistent with a metal sensitivity. Nickel is a common cause and is found in many objects, including jewelry, watches and snaps in clothing such as in jeans. The Köbner phenomenon describes a psoriatic response to trauma, most often observed in patients with psoriasis. Exposure to drugs can cause reactions that include dermatological findings. However, they tend to be much more diffuse. Eczema can present with localized irritation but doesn't account for the distribution in this patient. Psoriasis would occur in other skin distributions besides the isolated metal exposed areas. All of her findings are in areas directly exposed to metal.

Board Testing Point: Recognize metal sensitivity, especially nickel.

428. Answer: A

Answer: Prescribe tacrolimus cream (Protopic®) to be applied on the eczema.
Eczema is a recurrent inflammatory condition of the skin that typically begins in childhood and often persists into adulthood. Most treatments focus on control of the long-term symptoms and avoidance of exacerbating factors. Topical steroids are a useful adjunct in eczema therapy. Oral steroids, however, increase the potential of systemic side effects and do not improve the long-term course for eczematous patients. Strong topical steroids also have serious side effects. Immune modulators such as tacrolimus and pimecrolimus are approved for eczema treatment and do not affect the adrenocortical axis. Pruritus is a significant component of eczema and controlling the itch tends to improve the rash. Antihistamines can be very helpful, but H_2 blockers are not generally effective in this role. Patients with eczema display an increased incidence of skin infections, particularly with *S. Aureus*. Frequent soapy water increases the loss of vital skin emollients and tends to worsen the symptoms of eczema.

Board Testing Point: Summarize treatment strategies for eczema.

429. Answer: C

Answer: Carefully wash all clothing and tools from the work area to stop reinitiation of this rash.
Plants from the *Toxicodendron* genus, including poison oak, sumac, and ivy, are capable of causing significant symptoms. The plants produce an oleoresin that is absorbed by the skin and forms haptens, which are strong immune stimulants. The skin reaction involves pruritus and vesicular eruptions. Leukotriene inhibitors have no role in blocking or treating this process. The process is not contagious and the secretions do not contain free oleoresin. Therefore, the rash does not transmit from person to person by secretion contact. The resin, however, clings to tools and clothing for extended periods and can reinitiate a reaction with subsequent contact. Impetigo is a common complication of this process, and crusting of the secretions should prompt consideration for antibiotic therapy. In those situations, steroids should be used with clinical caution.

Board Testing Point: Control symptoms from exposure to toxicodendric plants.

430. Answer: A

Answer: Skin testing evaluates a broader range of allergic response mechanisms.
Skin testing follows well-prescribed techniques, and specially trained personnel are required to administer and evaluate the testing. Although skin testing is safe, it does cause significant dermal response. Since RAST testing requires only an IV blood draw, special collection training is not required, and it is less uncomfortable for the patient. Antihistamines can limit the reaction in skin testing but do not affect RAST results. RAST testing is limited to evaluation of IgE sensitivities, whereas skin testing evaluates a broader range of response mechanisms.

Board Testing Point: Analyze implications of testing for allergies.

431. Answer: E

Answer: Contact EMS for immediate transport to the nearest hospital.
An anaphylactic reaction to wasp and bee venom can be a life-threatening event and demands prompt intervention. The use of epinephrine can have a dramatic effect, but the half-life is short and the causative venom remains in the system for a much longer period. The use of epinephrine should be viewed as a therapeutic patch to maintain the patient until transport to an appropriate facility can occur. The other options are legitimate interventions, but are of much lower importance than prompt access to emergent medical care.

Board Testing Point: Recommend follow-up for anaphylaxis after treatment with epinephrine.

432. Answer: B

Answer: Systemic mastocytosis.
All of the processes described can present with flushing, palpitations, and edema. The lab values, however, are most consistent with systemic mastocytosis. In addition, the reddish-brown skin lesions represent urticaria pigmentosa, cutaneous clusters of mast cells. They are noted to cause urticaria and flushing when palpated, a reaction referred to as a Darier sign. A negative urine metanephrine and VMA test makes pheochromocytoma unlikely, and a normal 5-HIAA test likewise reduces the likelihood of a carcinoid tumor. A normal C1INH also makes angioedema unlikely. Tryptase is a protease found in mast cells, and elevated levels are found in anaphylactic reactions and conditions with increased mast cells, including mastocytosis.

Board Testing Point: Interpret the tryptase test to diagnose systemic mastocytosis in light of the appropriate history and physical exam.

433. Answer: B

Answer: Decrease in C1-inhibitor.
This is a case of hereditary angioedema, an autosomal dominant disorder associated with a decrease in C1-inhibitor with a secondarily decreased C4. Recurrent nonpitting edema is the norm, and each episode may last 1-2 days. The face and lips are commonly affected. In severe cases, laryngeal obstruction and GI manifestations may occur. It does not respond to epinephrine. None of the other choices fit this clinical profile.

Board Testing Point: Identify angioedema by history and associate the presentation with C1-inhibitor deficiency.

434. Answer: E

Answer: Recurrent and frequent infections with fungi, viruses, and protozoa.
Failure to thrive associated with diarrhea, recurrent viral infections, infection with opportunistic organisms, and fungal infections suggest an underlying T-cell immunodeficiency. Recurrent bacterial infection with encapsulated organisms such as pneumococci and *Haemophilus influenzae* are frequently observed with B-cell defects, as is a history of recurrent sinopulmonary infections. Susceptibility to infection with Giardia is also observed with B-cell deficiencies. Autoimmune diseases are more frequent with complement deficiencies.

Board Testing Point: Recognize which infections occur in patients with T-cell defects.

435. Answer: B

Answer: Serum IgA antibody level.
Patients with trisomy 21 are at increased risk of celiac disease caused by injury to the mucosa of the small intestine as a result of ingestion of gluten from wheat, rye, barely, and related grains. Serologic markers include both IgA antiendomysial and IgA tissue transglutaminase antibodies. Thus, it is essential to also order a serum IgA to document that the patient is not IgA deficient. IgA deficiency is more common in celiac disease, and such patients would therefore have false-negative results for the serologic markers described above. A small bowel biopsy is diagnostic when the patient is still ingesting gluten and shows villous atrophy and mucosal inflammation. Approximately 1 in 250-300 people in the United States, many of whom have not been diagnosed, have celiac disease. None of the other choices have a significant association with celiac disease.

Board Testing Point: Recognize the association of IgA deficiency with celiac disease.

436. Answer: D

Answer: Reassurance and suggest she take cool showers after exercise.
This patient suffers from hives induced by exercise and hot water, otherwise termed "cholinergic urticaria."
Because the classic features of cholinergic urticaria can be ascertained from her history (occurs after exercise,
associated with sweating or hot water), further workup need not be done. Urticaria is divided into "acute" and
"chronic" (occurs almost daily and lasts > 6 weeks). Acute urticaria can be due to several etiologies, including
medications, insect stings, latex allergy, food allergies, parasitic infections, contact allergens, ingested allergens
(such as radiocontrast medium) and reactions to certain physical conditions such as cold ("cold urticaria") and
heat ("cholinergic urticaria"). Chronic urticaria is more aggravating and worrisome and can be caused by systemic
diseases such as autoimmune states (lupus or thyroid dysfunction) and diseases of basophils and thrombin
formation. Complete blood counts, sedimentation rates, and complement levels are tests to distinguish the
etiology of urticaria in patients without an obvious cause. Cholinergic urticaria is frequently resistant to treatment
with antihistamines, although these drugs are the mainstay of treatment for cold urticaria.

Board Testing Point: Recognize cholinergic urticaria by history.

437. Answer: A

Answer: Ibuprofen 600 mg po and meperidine 50 mg IV.
This patient is experiencing a febrile, non-hemolytic transfusion reaction (FNHTR). Typical symptoms include
fever, chills, and subjective dyspnea without laboratory evidence of hemolysis. The hemolytic transfusion
reactions are more severe and can be associated with hypotension and acute renal failure. The DAT and
measurement of the free plasma hemoglobin are tests performed to assess whether acute hemolysis is occurring.
This patient is hemodynamically stable and has no objective evidence of pulmonary pathology; hence, he can be
managed conservatively with NSAIDS for fever and meperidine for severe chills.

Other transfusion reactions include:
Acute hemolytic transfusion reactions
Delayed hemolytic reactions
Anaphylactic reactions
Urticarial reactions
Transfusion-related acute lung injury

You should familiarize yourself with the characteristics, diagnostics, and treatment of each type of transfusion
reaction, since these are frequently tested concepts. He is having a transfusion reaction and does not require any of
the other interventions listed at this time.

Board Testing Point: Recognize a febrile, non-hemolytic transfusion reaction and prescribe appropriate
treatment.

438. Answer: D

Answer: Do not vaccinate him for MMR.
The occupational health department is indeed correct: a minimum of two doses of MMR vaccine are suggested for health care workers. However, since MMR is a live-virus vaccine, its administration is contraindicated in patients with advanced immunodeficiencies (including leukemia and lymphoma), CSF leaks, in patients receiving high-dose/long-term corticosteroids and in pregnancy. Were he to be HIV-negative, or have a higher CD4 count reflecting a better immune status, he would be a candidate for vaccination with MMR. His CD4 count of 11 cells/mm^3 categorizes him as severely immunocompromised. Varicella, another live-virus vaccine, is also contraindicated in immune-deficient patients. This patient cannot be safely vaccinated with MMR; the decision about whether or not he can work should be determined by the occupational health clinic where he is employed.

Board Testing Point: Recognize when the MMR vaccination is appropriate.

439. Answer: E

Answer: Hospitalize in the intensive care unit, and then contact an allergist to perform penicillin desensitization.
This classic Board question queries whether or not you know that penicillin G is the only drug with documented efficacy in treating syphilis in pregnancy. All pregnant patients, regardless of allergy, should receive penicillin for treatment. And, if a patient is truly allergic to beta-lactams, desensitization testing should be performed, and the patient should then be treated with penicillin.

The patient in question has latent syphilis of unknown duration, as determined by her becoming positive sometime in the past two years. She has no signs or symptoms of tertiary syphilis (cardiac, gummatous, or neurosyphilis), and her duration of infection is too short to be in the tertiary stage (considering she is HIV-negative).

Dosing of benzathine penicillin G 2.4 million units IM once is utilized in cases of primary and secondary syphilis. Tripling this dosage is used in patients with late, latent syphilis (infection for > 1 year) or in patients with latent syphilis of unknown duration. This patient is considered "syphilis of unknown duration" because her last test was 2 years ago, but you do not know when in the last two years she became infected: maybe > 1 year ago or maybe only 5 months ago. Azithromycin 2 g orally once is viable for primary and secondary syphilis in non-pregnant patients with penicillin allergy. Ceftriaxone has been recently studied and found effective in treatment of neurosyphilis in HIV+ patients. The 2006 MMWR STD Guidelines allow for use of ceftriaxone in the non-pregnant group for treatment of tertiary syphilis. However, ceftriaxone has not been studied in pregnancy. Penicillin G remains the drug of choice in this setting. Additionally, most patients with penicillin anaphylaxis will also react to the beta-lactam of the cephalosporins.

Board Testing Point: Synthesize a regimen for treatment of latent syphilis in the penicillin-allergic pregnant patient.

440. Answer: A

Answer: Isolated IgA deficiency.
Isolated IgA deficiency is the most common immunodeficiency and has an incidence between 1:600 and 1:800. People with this disorder have a normal or reduced number of B cells with surface IgA, but have an overabundance of immature cells that express both IgA and IgM. The problem is that it appears that the cells cannot secrete IgA effectively. Thus, there is a reduced amount of serum as well as secretory IgA. About 30-

40% of people with IgA deficiency have antibodies to IgA; thus if they get exposed to IgA (like in blood products or IVIG) they will have anaphylaxis. None of the other listed choices would result in an anaphylactic reaction with blood products.

Board Testing Point: Recognize IgA deficiency in the face of exposure to blood products.

441. Answer: B

Answer: Serum immunoglobulins.
He most likely has immunoglobulin A deficiency. IgA serves as the first line of defense against infections of the respiratory tract as well as infections of the GI and GU tracts. IgA deficiency is really fairly common! 1/ 600 individuals of European ancestry will have the deficiency. People with IgA deficiency are usually healthy, but they may have frequent episodes of upper respiratory tract infections, bronchiectasis, and chronic diarrhea. They are also more prone to allergies, asthma, and other autoimmune disorders. HIV infection is much less likely, particularly with his sexual history listed and his problems stemming since childhood. This is not *Mycoplasma*, so cold agglutinins are not indicated, and he has not had any infections with organisms that would make terminal complement deficiency likely. Serum protein electrophoresis will not provide any useful data in this patient.

Board Testing Point: Recognize the clinical findings of IgA deficiency.

DERMATOLOGY

442. Answer: D

Answer: Prescribe benzoyl peroxide for both comedolytic and antiseptic activity.
Benzoyl peroxide has both comedolytic and antiseptic activity. Topical clindamycin has antiseptic activity but no significant comedolytic activity. Studies have demonstrated that diet does not directly affect sebum levels, but topical oils and greases may increase pore occlusion and worsen acne. Retinoids are prescribed to females of reproductive age only after topical therapy fails to control breakouts since they are known teratogens. Sexually active females must be managed with aggressive contraception (at least 2 methods) while taking oral retinoids.

Board Testing Point: Knowledge of acne treatments and use of oral retinoids in women of reproductive age.

443. Answer: B

Answer: Malignancy of the gastrointestinal tract.
He has seborrheic keratoses, which are common benign macules, papules, and plaques typically affecting individuals over the age of 30. They appear as waxy stuck-on lesions found anywhere except the palms, soles, and mucous membranes. The rare sign of Leser-Trélat or eruptive seborrheic keratoses is associated with an internal malignancy. While the seborrheic keratoses associated with this sign are benign, their striking proliferation or rapid increase in number and size is highly suggestive of a malignant adenocarcinoma. He is not at increased risk for melanoma or squamous cell carcinoma.

Board Testing Point: Associate the need for gastrointestinal evaluation in a setting of rapid development of seborrheic keratoses.

444. Answer: A

Answer: Pityriasis rosea.
This question aims at identifying the etiology of a papulosquamous eruption using only clues from the history and physical examination. The word papulosquamous suggests a "rash" that is firm, raised-up, and scaly. All of options can cause papulosquamous eruptions, but the history and PE should help you identify the etiology. Based on the history and the negative RPR, secondary syphilis can be excluded with excellent reliability. Tinea versicolor will have a KOH prep that shows the typical "spaghetti and meatball" appearance of *Malassezia furfur*. While erythema chronicum migrans due to Lyme disease rarely can be associated with multiple secondary lesions, the rash is described as erythematous with central clearing (more of a "target") and is infrequently associated with scaling. Psoriasis classically involves the knees and elbows, at minimum, and is extremely pruritic. Pityriasis rosea is a papulosquamous rash characterized by the onset of a "herald patch," which precedes the disseminated eruption of plaques. The rash varies from non-pruritic to severely pruritic. KOH smears demonstrate no fungal elements, and the RPR should be negative. The rash usually will spontaneously resolve in three months; but if the rash remains, a biopsy should be performed to exclude parapsoriasis. Treatment for pityriasis rosea is supportive with moisturizers and antihistamines. Sometimes, the sun helps the lesions to be less pruritic.

Board Testing Point: Recognize pityriasis rosea as the etiology of a papulosquamous rash using history, physical exam, and laboratory clues.

445. Answer: B

Answer: Esophageal dysmotility.
The patient in question demonstrates CREST syndrome, a variant of scleroderma (sustained abnormal synthesis and deposition of collagen). The picture is showing a telangiectasia. Patients with scleroderma are now classified according to organ involvement and antibody profile:

- Limited cutaneous systemic sclerosis (LcSSc)
- Diffuse cutaneous systemic sclerosis (DcSSc)
- Systemic sclerosis sine scleroderma

LcSSc frequently presents as the CREST syndrome (a mnemonic employed to describe the clinical manifestations of **c**alcinosis, **R**aynaud phenomenon, **e**sophageal dysmotility, **s**clerodactyly, and **t**elangiectasia). Prior to development of true skin thickening, patients can present with non-pitting edema and erythema of the extremities. Disease limited to skin on the extremities is often not as severe as disease that becomes diffuse, involving multiple organ systems. Interestingly, antibody profiles seem to prognosticate what future organs will become involved. Patients with only anti-centromere antibodies tend to have limited, peripheral manifestations (i.e. CREST), as opposed to patients who have anti-SCL-70 antibodies, who suffer from diffuse organ involvement including interstitial fibrosis and renal crisis.

Board Testing Point: Diagnose CREST syndrome, and associate anti-centromere antibodies with this limited form of scleroderma.

446. Answer: E

Answer: *Mycoplasma pneumoniae*.
Erythema multiforme consists of well-defined lesions varying from annular to target shape. Palms and soles are frequently involved. The target or iris-shaped lesions are pathognomonic for erythema multiforme. The lesions may also be edematous or bullous. It is caused by many infectious and noninfectious etiologies; mycoplasma and herpes simplex are commonly associated. While erythema migrans can present as multiple lesions, the history in this patient is not adequate to make a diagnosis of Lyme disease, and the upper respiratory features clearly point to *Mycoplasma pneumoniae* as an etiology. Secondary syphilis does not commonly present as target lesions, and this patient denies sexual activity. Adenovirus and hepatitis C rarely would cause these types of lesions.

Board Testing Point: Recognize the association between infectious agents and erythema multiforme.

447. Answer: C

Answer: The causative agent resides in the dorsal root ganglion of the spinal cord.
Childhood varicella or chickenpox is caused by the varicella-zoster virus. The picture is showing a Tzanck smear, which shows multinucleated giant cells. These can occur with any herpes virus, including varicella, but only varicella virus is responsible for zoster infection. Once you get this childhood disease, the virus remains in the dorsal root ganglion of the spinal cord and resurfaces as zoster when immunity is low. Herpes simplex virus infections (type 1 and 2) present as grouped vesicles on an erythematous base. Dermatomal distribution is very characteristic of zoster. It is an endogenous infection requiring that the patient have varicella first before developing zoster. One attack usually confers immunity.

Board Testing Point: Discern the etiology of herpes zoster and where the virus is dormant.

448. Answer: B

Answer: Chronic herpetic ulceration.
The retrovirus associated with being HIV-positive causes waning of immunity. While any of the choices could cause ulcerations, by far the most likely etiology is herpes stomatitis. If there is no response after empiric treatment, then other possibilities should be considered.

Board Testing Point: Recognize the association of HIV infection with herpetic ulcerations of the mouth.

449. Answer: D

Answer: Human herpesvirus type VIII (HHV-8).
There is still controversy about whether Kaposi sarcoma is a malignant vascular endothelial proliferation (therefore, a true neoplasm) or only a virally induced endothelial hyperplasia (and thus not truly a cancer). The virus found frequently associated with AIDS-related epidemic KS is HHV-8. The other viruses listed are not associated with Kaposi sarcoma.

Board Testing Point: Remember the most likely etiology of Kaposi sarcoma.

450. Answer: C

Answer: Diabetes.
There are numerous causes of exfoliative erythroderma since it is a final common pathway for numerous disease processes. To date, however, there have been no reported cases secondary to diabetes. All of the other choices can cause exfoliative erythroderma.

Board Testing Point: Reproduce a differential diagnosis for exfoliative dermatitis.

451. Answer: A

Answer: Nodules of condylomata acuminata.
Squamous cell carcinoma has been reported in large warts of the genital area. It is thought that the human papilloma virus, which causes warts, may act as a cocarcinogen, causing the development of squamous cell carcinoma. No neoplasms have been associated with the other options listed.

Board Testing Point: Recognize the association of human papilloma virus with the development of squamous cell carcinoma and which population is most often affected.

452. Answer: D

Answer: Avoid a sunburn.
Since gene re-arrangement is not yet available to avoid the development of malignant melanoma, the American Academy of Dermatology recommends using a sunscreen with a SPF of 30, wearing a wide-brim hat, avoiding the sun in the summer between 10 AM and 4 PM, and avoiding sunburns. So far, increased sleep and broccoli consumption have not been shown to reduce the risk of melanoma.

Board Testing Point: Understand that the largest risk factor for melanoma is previous sunburn.

453. Answer: D

Answer: Tinea versicolor.
Tinea versicolor, sometimes called pityriasis versicolor, is a chronic, asymptomatic scaling dermatosis caused by an overgrowth of *Pityrosporum orbiculare* (also known as *P. ovale* and *Malassezia furfur*). It is commonly seen in young adults, and the incidence tapers off during the fifth and sixth decades. While it commonly presents with hypopigmented perifollicular macules, it can also be seen as hyperpigmented scaling macules and patches. A positive KOH preparation is a diagnostic test that separates it from the other choices. On the KOH prep you expect to see a "spaghetti and meatballs" pattern. None of the other choices are due to fungi.

Board Testing Point: Diagnose tinea versicolor.

454. Answer: E

Answer: Shave biopsy of the lesion for pathology.
This lesion is a basal cell carcinoma, the most common form of skin cancer. Basal cell carcinomas (BCCs) are malignant tumors that are locally aggressive, destructive, and invasive but rarely metastatic. They are most common in fair skinned persons with chronic sun exposure and are generally seen in older adults.   Rarely seen in brown- and black-skinned individuals, the lesions can be pearly and nodular with extensive telangectasias or ulcerative. Frequently, lesions are a combination of these two forms.   These tumors are most commonly treated surgically, although cryotherapy is an acceptable form of treatment for superficial multicentric BCCs. None of the other choices would be the first step. Remember, when presented with a suspicious skin lesion, it is almost always best to biopsy.

Board Testing Point: Construct a management plan for obvious basal cell carcinoma.

455. Answer: A

Answer: Observation only.
The described lesion is a dermatofibroma. Dermatofibromas may be erythematous, tan, or hyperpigmented. They are dome-shaped papules with a firm consistency and are seen on legs, arms, and trunk. The "dimple sign" is quite specific, with central depression secondary to lateral pressure that is common with dermatofibroma. While not considered a marker of internal problems, it is thought that everyone has at least one. The lesion has no features concerning for a malignant neoplasm, nor does the patient complain of symptoms worrisome for metastatic disease. Biopsy of this lesion is not necessary if the classic features are present, including the dimple sign (so this is one of those cases when biopsy is not the correct answer). None of the other tests would be needed since this is a benign condition requiring no further workup.

Board Testing Point: Interpret a "dimple sign" when associated with an asymptomatic nodular lesion on the extremities that is consistent with a dermatofibroma.

456. Answer: C

Answer: Nailfold telangiectasia.
Systemic lupus erythematosus (SLE) can present with a "malar rash," referred to as "butterfly" in type. Usually, it is bright red in color and sharply defined with slight edema and scaling. Sandpaper truncal rash is most commonly seen with *S. pyogenes* infection (scarlet fever). In SLE, palmar erythema (not exfoliation), nailfold telangiectasia,

and photosensitivity can be seen. Acrosclerosis is frequently seen in systemic sclerosis accompanied by necrosis and ulcerations of fingertips, but is not seen in SLE.

Board Testing Point: Recognize nailfold telangiectasias as a finding associated with systemic lupus erythematosus.

457. Answer: D

Answer: Dermatitis herpetiformis.

Dermatitis herpetiformis is a chronic, recurrent vesicular eruption (often on an erythematous base) in a strikingly bilateral pattern, usually associated with a gluten-sensitive enteropathy. Often, there are no systemic symptoms related to the GI tract, and the rash is present in isolation. Ingestion of iodides can precipitate the rash development, because iodide complexes to IgA in the same way as the gluten, subsequently depositing in the skin. Dermatopathology reveals IgA deposits in the tips of the dermal papillae. A gluten-free diet helps in management; daily dapsone also helps some individuals. Secondary syphilis and guttate psoriasis are associated with papulosquamous eruptions, not vesicular rashes. Varicella zoster eruptions are vesicular but do not have the striking bilateral symmetry as seen with this condition. The etiology of dermatitis herpetiformis is not herpes, in spite of the name. Eczema would not present in this fashion.

Board Testing Point: Associate a recurrent, bilateral vesicular rash with gluten-sensitive enteropathy.

458. Answer: D

Answer: Fluorinated steroids.

Topical steroids may initially improve acne by decreasing the erythema and inflammation. One of the side effects of topical steroids, especially the fluorinated ones, is that they produce an acneiform eruption. All of the other medications listed are accepted acne treatment.

Board Testing Point: Recognize acceptable acne treatments.

459. Answer: D

Answer: Malignant melanoma.

The decision as to whether or not a lesion is a melanoma can be expedited by using the ABCD mnemonic. The A stands for asymmetry, B for border (irregular), C for color (change), and D for diameter (increasing). Insert how the photograph reflects abnormalities in ABCD. Seborrheic keratoses appear after age 30 and have a plaque-like, warty consistency; they often appear as if they were "stuck on" the skin. They can sometimes be mistaken for melanoma when very large. Junctional melanocytic nevocellular nevi are round, smooth and flat and do not have malignant potential. Keratoacanthomas arise on the face, usually, with a dome shape and a central keratinaceous plug. Breast cancer only rarely metastasizes to the skin. This lesion is more likely to be melanoma.

Board Testing Point: Remember the ABCD mnemonic for the Boards. They are likely to give you a lesion that has the 4 components and you'll need to recognize the lesion as suspicious.

460. Answer: D

Answer: Topical liquid nitrogen and 5% 5-fluorouracil cream.
The lesions in this case are classic solar keratoses (also termed "actinic keratoses"). The lesions are dry with adherent scale on the exposed skin surfaces. In the context of obvious over-exposure to the sun, these lesions are easy to distinguish. They appear similar to seborrheic keratoses, but they do not have the erythematous base; and actinic keratoses are often only on sun-exposed surfaces. Actinic keratoses are precursor lesions to squamous cell carcinoma. These lesions typically remain for years unless they are treated. Treatment consists of topical application of liquid nitrogen followed by topical chemotherapy. Counseling to avoid sun exposure is essential. Botulism toxin injections will not affect actinic keratoses. Ketoconazole cream and topical steroids will not affect them either. HIV does not predispose to this condition. These lesions can be diagnosed clinically and do not require biopsy except in cases where they resemble lesions of discoid lupus erythematosus.

Board Testing Point: Manage a case of actinic keratoses.

461. Answer: D

Answer: Atopic dermatitis.
These common hypopigmented patches are frequently found on the face and referred to as pityriasis alba. They can be markers of atopic dermatitis, asthma, or allergic rhinoconjunctivitis. They can also be seen without associated disease. The pathogenesis is unknown, and resolution occurs spontaneously with age. None of the other conditions are associated with pityriasis alba.

Board Testing Point: Associate the rash of pityriasis alba with atopic dermatitis.

462. Answer: D

Answer: Turn the patient every 2 hours.
This patient has a stage I pressure ulcer. Stage I ulcers have intact skin with nonblanchable erythema. Stage II ulcers involve the epidermidis, dermis, or both. Stage III ulcers involve the full thickness of the skin and extend into the subcutaneous tissue. Stage IV involves muscle, bone, and associated supporting tissues.

Treatment for all pressure sores involves minimizing pressure and keeping the surrounding area clean. Adequate nutrition is also very important. Stage I ulcers may be treated by rotating the patient every 2 hours to reduce the pressure; in many instances, this is the most effective therapy. Stages II-IV require more intense therapy, all of which are meant to keep the wound clean and moist. For these later stages, dressing changes should be as infrequent as possible to minimize disruption of reepithelialization. Stage III and IV require surgical debridement. Air beds are also useful for Stage III and IV wounds. Doughnut cushions are ineffective and should be avoided because they cause venous congestion and edema.

Board Testing Point: Recognize the findings of a Stage I pressure ulcer and understand how best to treat it.

463. Answer: C

Answer: Reassure the patient that the condition is temporary.
The patient described has telogen effluvium, a common form of noninflammatory diffuse hair loss. It often follows an illness; in this case, infectious mononucleosis, which triggers an abnormally high number of anagen (growing) hairs to switch over to the telogen (resting) phase. Several months following the illness, diffuse brisk telogen hair loss occurs. Although distressing, this indicates the end of the process. The patient can be reassured that new anagen hair growth will result in the return of pre-telogen effluvium hair length during the next several months. None of the other therapies listed are necessary or indicated.

Board Testing Point: Recognize telogen effluvium as a common cause of hair loss after illness or stress.

OB / GYN

464. Answer: D

Answer: Continue the same immunosuppressives, but stop the losartan and atorvastatin.
This case focuses on medications during pregnancy. Angiotensin-converting enzyme inhibitors and angiotensin-receptor blockers are contraindicated in pregnancy, as are statins; therefore, they should be discontinued in patients planning pregnancy, or if they are taking these medicines and become pregnant. Diuretics should generally not be used for treatment of hypertension in pregnancy. The preferred agents are methyldopa and hydralazine, but labetalol is also safe. With regard to transplant medications, the calcineurin inhibitors, cyclosporine, tacrolimus, and prednisone are acceptable in pregnancy. Azathioprine has been used safely in pregnancy during transplantation but still carries a Category D warning. There is inadequate information available regarding mycophenolate; therefore, her current immunosuppressive medications are acceptable, but she needs to discontinue the losartan and atorvastatin. There is no need to increase her prednisone just because of her pregnant state.

Board Testing Point: Recognize that angiotensin-converting enzyme inhibitors and statins are contraindicated in pregnancy.

465. Answer: B

Answer: Folate.
Good nutrition with adequate levels of all vitamins and nutrients is important during pregnancy. Folate, however, has specifically been identified as an important adjunct in reducing the risk of neural tube defects. To be most effective, the supplements should be started before conception and continued throughout the course of the pregnancy. The other vitamins listed are important, but folate is the most important in early fetal development.

Board Testing Point: Prescribe folate in early pregnancy to prevent neural tube defects.

466. Answer: B

Answer: Polycystic ovarian syndrome.
The control of menstrual cycles is regulated by the interplay of FSH and LH on the ovaries, and estrogen and progesterone on the uterine lining. Measurement of these hormones is helpful in determining the specific etiology for a menstrual abnormality. With polycystic ovarian syndrome (PCOS), the ovaries become increasingly resistant to stimulation for ovulation. PCOS is associated with increased circulating estrogens, as well as increased androgens. The increased estrogens suppress FSH release, and the ovulatory failure results in increased levels of LH.

Premature ovarian failure arises when the ovaries no longer respond to follicular stimulation. Due to the diminished response, the estrogen levels fall, and the FSH and LH levels rise.

Prolactinoma increases prolactin levels that serve as inhibitors to the release of FSH and LH and, subsequently, to decreased estrogen levels. Anorexia nervosa also typically demonstrates decreased LH and decreased FSH and decreased estrogen.

Asherman syndrome results from damage to the endometrial portion of the uterus that interferes with the development of the proliferative phase of the menstrual cycle. The hormonal axis remains intact with normal LH, FSH, and estrogen levels and continues to cycle despite the lack of endometrial response.

Board Testing Point: Interpret hormone laboratories and diagnose polycystic ovary syndrome as an etiology of amenorrhea.

467. Answer: E

Answer: Tetanus, influenza.
This patient should have the influenza vaccine and an updated tetanus booster. She should not be given a varicella vaccine or an MMR vaccine because the vaccine contains live, attenuated viruses, and she is pregnant. (She has likely already had varicella, in spite of failing to recall being infected. Often, cases of true varicella are sub-clinical and unrecognized by children and their parents. Obtaining anti-varicella antibodies would be useful in determining if she is truly at risk.) Whether to administer MMR to a pregnant patient is a favorite board question.

Board Testing Point: Avoid prescribing live-virus vaccines in pregnancy.

468. Answer: B

Answer: Acute tubular necrosis.
This patient developed acute oliguric renal failure following a spontaneous septic abortion. These patients do have volume losses; but if she had pre-renal azotemia only, she should have responded to IV fluids and transfusions. Preeclampsia is excluded because her ARF occurred at 12 weeks; preeclampsia should rarely be considered before 20-week gestation. Preeclampsia is usually not associated with severe renal failure unless the patient also has the HELLP syndrome. This patient has normal platelets which is inconsistent with HELLP.

In this patient, there is no indication or reason to suspect rhabdomyolysis. Not only would the CPK be elevated, but one would expect few RBCs with a positive dipstick for blood. Historically, renal cortical necrosis is described in obstetric catastrophe, and this setting would be appropriate. However, this disorder causes prolonged, severe oliguric and even anuric renal failure that may eventually recover after many months, usually leaving persistent renal dysfunction. This patient has acute tubular necrosis. The features that are consistent with this diagnosis are the clinical setting of hypotension and sepsis, and a urinalysis with granular casts.

Board Testing Point: Interpret basic metabolic tests and diagnose acute tubular necrosis in pregnancy.

469. Answer: A

Answer: Prompt delivery of her child.
Preeclampsia with hypertension and significant proteinuria is a serious complication of pregnancy and can progress to convulsions and maternal demise. The association of hemolytic anemia, elevated liver enzymes and low platelets is described as the HELLP syndrome. Its exact mechanism is under investigation, but plasmapheresis has no role in its management. Transfusions may be required to stabilize the patient for delivery, but do not improve the renal or hepatic components. Steroids may accelerate the maturation of the fetus for delivery, but do not treat the underlying pathology involved in preeclampsia. The treatment for both preeclampsia and for HELLP syndrome is the prompt termination of the pregnancy and supportive care for the mother.

Board Testing Point: Interpret basic laboratory tests and integrate them with a history to diagnose pre-eclampsia; recommend treatment.

470. Answer: A

Answer: Topical estrogen.
Postmenopausal atrophy of the vaginal mucosa can lead to dysuria, dyspareunia, and pruritus. The findings of atrophic vaginal mucosa with easy irritation and parabasal cells on wet mount are consistent with estrogen deficiency. There is no evidence of gonorrhea (ceftriaxone), chlamydia (doxycycline), *Trichomonas* or *Gardnerella* (metronidazole), or significant urinary tract infection. There was no discharge on pelvic examination or hyphae or pseudo hyphae noted on wet mount (clotrimazole). Low-frequency topical estrogen is effective at restoring vaginal mucosa, which can limit atrophic symptoms and can also reduce the incidence of infections. Limited use is a relatively safe method for local hormone replacement.

Board Testing Point: Recognize the findings of postmenopausal vaginal atrophy.

471. Answer: B

Answer: Positive urine pregnancy test.
Emergency hormonal contraceptive intervention must be instituted prior to the implantation of the fertilized ovum. In this condition, both urine and serum pregnancy tests must be negative. A positive pregnancy test indicates that a pregnancy is already established, and emergent dosing of hormonal contraception is not effective. Now, if a woman takes the "morning after" pill, will it harm the developing fetus? No, but it will also likely not be effective in terminating the pregnancy. Oral retinoids are highly teratogenic agents, and their use at the time of conception is a strong indication to terminate an impending pregnancy. Inadequate compliance with a contraceptive regimen is the most common reason to consider emergent contraception. It should prompt further encouragement at adherence to long-term family planning but is not a contraindication to emergent contraception.

Board Testing Point: Recognize that the presence of an implanted fertilized ovum is a contraindication for emergent hormonal contraception.

472. Answer: D

Answer: Results of bone density scans performed by different techniques are difficult to directly compare.
Bone density studies can be helpful to document and follow levels of osteoporosis. However, there is significant variation between the different techniques, which makes comparison among different studies very problematic. Routine radiographic studies are insensitive at demonstrating mild-to-moderate osteoporosis. The results of bone density studies are reported as a t-score and a z-score. The t-score is based on comparison to sex-matched standards based on results of bone density norms of young healthy adults. The z-score is based on a comparison to a sex-matched standard based on age-matched peers. Positive levels are higher than the mean and negative values are lower than the mean.

Board Testing Point: Interpret a bone density scan in a patient at risk for osteoporosis.

473. Answer: A

Answer: Uterine/adnexal tenderness OR cervical motion tenderness.
Empiric treatment of pelvic inflammatory disease is recommended if minimal criteria are identified and, in this case, there is uterine or adnexal tenderness OR cervical motion tenderness. The other options, except for the previous documented infection within the past 3 months, represent additional criteria that support the diagnosis of

pelvic inflammatory disease. However, they are not diagnostic for pelvic inflammatory disease, just suggestive. The diagnosis of previous infection does not play a role in the evaluation or treatment of a new infection.

Board Testing Point: For the Boards, recognize that there is a VERY low threshold for initiating therapy for pelvic inflammatory disease.

474. Answer: B

Answer: Tubo-ovarian abscess in the differential diagnosis.
Patients with pelvic inflammatory disease should be hospitalized under the following circumstances:

- Cannot exclude a surgical emergency
- Pregnancy
- Failure of oral treatment
- Unable to cooperate with or tolerate outpatient therapy
- Severe symptoms such as high fever, nausea, or vomiting
- Suspected tubo-ovarian abscess

None of the other choices increase a patient's risk for complication and therefore do not warrant hospitalization by themselves.

Board Testing Point: Identify situations where hospitalization for treatment of PID is warranted.

475. Answer: E

Answer: Seizure disorder.
Several anticonvulsants including phenytoin, carbamazepine, and valproic acid are associated with an embryopathy that includes facial and limb abnormalities as well as spinal dysraphism. It is still unclear whether the teratogenic effect is a result of the seizure disorder or treatment with anticonvulsants. Infants born to mothers with a history of a seizure disorder are at increased risk of congenital anomalies, even if the mother is not treated with anticonvulsants during her pregnancy. Of note: Infants of mothers treated with lithium for bipolar disease during pregnancy are at an increased risk of Ebstein anomaly. Medications used to treat the other conditions during a pregnancy would not result in this type of embryopathy.

Board Testing Point: Recognize that anticonvulsants such as carbamazepine and valproic acid are associated with embryopathy during pregnancy.

476. Answer: D

Answer: Perihepatitis.
She most likely has pelvic inflammatory disease due to *N. gonorrhoeae* or *Chlamydia* associated with perihepatitis or Fitz-Hugh-Curtis syndrome. During menses, *N. gonorrhoeae* and/or *Chlamydia* may ascend into the peritoneum through the fallopian tubes and seed the liver capsule causing a perihepatitis. This often presents with right upper quadrant pain associated with signs and symptoms of upper and lower genital tract infection. In an effort to provide prompt and efficient treatment to prevent further infectious complications and decrease the risk of sterility, hospitalization and treatment with intravenous antibiotics is indicated.

Board Testing Point: Diagnose Fitz-Hugh Curtis syndrome (perihepatitis) based on history and physical exam.

OPHTHAMOLOGY

477. Answer: E

Answer: Hospital admission for intravenous acyclovir at a dose of 10 mg/kg.
This is a case of reactive herpes zoster ophthalmicus in an immunosuppressed patient, as manifested by classic vesicular lesions in a dermatomal distribution (the first branch of the trigeminal nerve, V1). V1 innervates the forehead, the tip of the nose, the eyelids, much of the orbit and corneal sensation; lesions presenting in this distribution suggest that virus may also be reactivating in the eye, even if lesions are not visible. If patients have any ocular signs or symptoms, the eye is assumed to be involved. In very immunosuppressed persons, distinguishing lesions of varicella zoster from herpes simplex may prove difficult, since HSV can also reactivate in a dermatomal distribution. Corneal ulcers may have distinguishing characteristics but, in patients with early ocular involvement, differences between HSV and VZV may not be appreciable. Zoster ophthalmicus is a sight-threatening condition, and immediate treatment is essential, including ophthalmologic evaluation. Higher doses of acyclovir are required to inhibit replication of varicella compared to HSV, and both zoster and HSV have a tendency to disseminate and infect the central nervous system, especially in immunocompromised patients. Hence, dermatomal vesicular rashes in these populations should be considered as varicella. If the eye is involved, or if the infection includes multiple dermatomes, the outbreak should be treated with higher doses of intravenous acyclovir.

Board Testing Point: Recognize the seriousness of zoster involvement in the VI distribution.

478. Answer: A

Answer: Acute angle-closure glaucoma.
This is a case of a sight-threatening emergency. Diagnosis of this form of glaucoma requires:

2/3 symptoms	Ocular pain Nausea/vomiting History of blurring with halos
3/5 signs	Elevated intraocular pressure (> 21 mm Hg) Conjunctival injection Corneal epithelial edema Mid-dilated nonreactive pupil Shallower chamber in the presence of occlusion

The patient's daughter clearly has a secondary bacterial infection of the conjunctiva as a result of a viral infection, but the father does not have the same symptoms. His symptoms are worrisome for an ophthalmologic emergency: a red, painful eye with reduced visual acuity. This form of glaucoma may present with headache and nausea/vomiting, leading some practitioners to diagnose patients with migraine headaches, thus potentially causing permanent vision loss. In the patient's history, he is describing blurry vision and the presence of halos, none of which are present in simple adenoviral conjunctivitis. Sympathomimetic medications, such as pseudoephedrine, can precipitate acute angle closure. Cluster headaches are not associated with eye pain or vision disturbances, only excessive tearing and headache. Fusarium keratitis is seen in the setting of an ocular foreign body with corneal ulceration, or recently, with the usage of certain contact lens solutions and poor lens hygiene. Subarachnoid hemorrhages may cause headache but do not cause eye redness, pain, or vision loss.

Board Testing Point: Recognize acute angle-closure glaucoma, an acute ophthalmologic emergency, and distinguishing it from other potential causes of eye pain through history and physical examination.

479. Answer: D

Answer: Emergent referral to an ophthalmologist.
This is a case of acute angle-closure glaucoma. His symptoms are worrisome for a sight-threatening emergency: a red, painful eye with reduced visual acuity. Patients with this form of glaucoma sometimes present with headache and nausea/vomiting, leading some practitioners to diagnose patients with migraine headaches. In the patient's history, he is describing blurry vision and the presence of halos, none of which are present in simple adenoviral conjunctivitis. Sympathomimetic medications, such as pseudoephedrine, can precipitate acute angle closure. The treatment is urgent reduction of the elevated intraocular pressure by an ophthalmologist to prevent permanent vision loss.

Board Testing Point: Recognize acute angle-closure glaucoma and the need for urgent referral to an ophthalmologist.

480. Answer: D

Answer: Reassurance with continued temporary abstinence from contact lens wear.
This is a case of viral conjunctivitis, or "pink eye" as described by upper respiratory tract symptoms and a slightly erythematous, but non-painful, left eye. The lack of severe pain and acuity or motion impairment is evidence that the infection is limited to the conjunctiva. This condition is often caused by a common respiratory virus, such as adenovirus, and commonly self-resolves. Antibiotics are not indicated in cases of viral conjunctivitis when no secondary bacterial infection is present. Contact lenses should not be worn when the eye is experiencing infection. While occult foreign bodies occur, this patient has a classic history of upper respiratory symptoms preceding her eye complaints, making viral conjunctivitis the most likely etiology.

Board Testing Point: Identification and management of viral conjunctivitis.

481. Answer: A

Answer: Bilateral blindness.
Elements of the history, when taken in concert, suggest this patient is suffering from temporal arteritis (also known as giant cell arteritis). She fits the common profile (> 70 years and female), and she demonstrates the most common complaints: headache, jaw claudication, and vision disturbances. Her headache, while unusual in characterization, is due to inflammation of the temporal artery. Systemic symptoms of fatigue, anorexia, and weight loss are fairly common. Giant cell arteritis should be suspected in any female over the age of 70 who complains of head or scalp discomfort; prompt diagnosis requires a high index of suspicion. 50% of patients with temporal arteritis initially complain of vision changes, and bilateral blindness occurs in up to 50% of those who are untreated.

Board Testing Point: Recognize temporal arteritis and the risk of blindness in this condition if untreated.

482. Answer: B

Answer: Chest radiograph.
She has the classic clinical history and physical examination findings for sarcoidosis. She is an African-American female with lung involvement, anterior uveitis, and arthritis. A chest radiograph would confirm her lung findings. Over 90% of cases of sarcoid uveitis have abnormal chest radiographs at presentation. The arthritis of sarcoid is usually symmetric and involving joints of the lower extremities. Although Lyme disease can also cause an

anterior chamber uveitis and arthritis, pulmonary findings are not present in Lyme disease. Screening Lyme titers are often false positive and should not be considered as proof of diagnosis in their own right. No history of travel to endemic areas drastically reduces the pre-test probability of Lyme disease in this patient. Tuberculosis and inflammatory bowel disease also cause anterior chamber uveitis, but this patient's lung findings and negative review of systems are not consistent with those diagnoses.

Board Testing Point: Recognize sarcoidosis with anterior uveitis as a primary presentation.

483. Answer: E

Answer: Referral to an ophthalmologist for evaluation today.
This is a case of retinal detachment, and this patient's underlying immune deficiency is not related to the current clinical problem. New-onset floaters and flashing lights are considered signs of retinal detachment until proven otherwise. This patient's risk factors for retinal detachment are male sex, age 40-60, history of myopia, and recent trauma to the head. Note, however, that retinal detachments due to paint ball trauma are now seen much more frequently in younger age groups (teens, especially). Retinal detachment is one of the most time-sensitive ophthalmologic emergencies, and patients should be counseled to get emergent attention, regardless of their personal plans, and even when their vision is not yet impaired. Changes in visual acuity from retinal detachment occur late. Valganciclovir is given for cytomegalovirus retinitis, of which this patient has no symptoms and for which he is not at risk given his CD4 count. Sumatriptan succinate is given for migraine headaches. Since this patient has not developed a headache, the flashing lights should not be considered migraine-associated scotoma.

The key aspects of this question were the acute change and the need for emergent evaluation by an ophthalmologist. You really didn't need to figure out what the etiology of his problem was, just that he needed to be seen by the specialist right away. This is common in Board "eye" questions. The Boards know that we as general internists really don't deal much with these emergent types of problems, and in general it is usually best to refer these quickly if something "is not right" with the patient. Now don't get upset if you are well versed in this area! Congrats to you, but a majority of internists do not feel comfortable with these types of presentations and the Boards know that, so they give us the "easy out" of calling in our specialist colleague quickly. This in reality is the best thing to do for our patients! ☺

Board Testing Point: Recognize of symptoms of retinal detachment, an ophthalmologic emergency.

484. Answer: C

Answer: HIV ELISA test.
The weight loss, nebulous skin rashes, and vision changes suggest a diagnosis of HIV infection and AIDS. The funduscopic findings of exudates and scattered hemorrhages ("pizza-pie eye") suggest bilateral, severe cytomegalovirus infection and a profound degree of immunodeficiency. Once HIV infection is established, and the CD4 count is quantified to reveal a severe degree of immune deficiency, CMV retinitis can be diagnosed solely on the basis of history and physical examination. Empiric treatment can then be initiated. Valganciclovir is considered the treatment of choice for CMV retinitis because of its superior bioavailability and ease of dosing when compared with traditional ganciclovir. CMV disease in HIV+ patients is a reactivation-illness; patients harbor CMV for most of their lives and only when their immune system is damaged do they manifest disease. IgM antibodies rise and fall throughout our lifetimes and do not correlate with active infection of CMV. An absent IgG antibody, however, would indicate that this particular patient had never been exposed to CMV. The lack of an IgG antibody, however, should not dissuade you from making a diagnosis of CMV in a profoundly immune-suppressed patient with classic clinical findings. Syphilis can cause disease of the eye, especially in HIV+ patients, but the presentation is a granulomatous iridis or anterior/posterior/pan-uveitis. These conditions

have a markedly different appearance and symptom profile from retinitis. *Bartonella henselae* can cause chronic low-grade bacteremia and bacillary angiomatosis/peliosis in HIV+ patients, but is not associated with eye disease.

Board Testing Point: Patients with undiagnosed immune deficiency on the Boards will frequently have vague symptoms that you must "put together" using non-specific findings and clues. In this example, CMV retinitis presents as an AIDS-defining illness in a young man with weight loss, skin rashes, and vision changes.

---

485. Answer: B

Answer: Non-Hodgkin lymphoma.
Sjögren syndrome is an auto-immune disorder associated with an abnormal proliferation of lymphocytes and tissue infiltration. While this disorder can be associated with other auto-immune diseases, such as rheumatoid arthritis and systemic lupus erythematosus, this patient does not have signs or symptoms of those disorders at this time. Hence, her diagnosis would be primary Sjögren syndrome. Universal consensus does not exist for specific diagnostic criteria for Sjögren's, but these features are highly associated:

- Symptoms of reduced tear production
- Symptoms of reduced saliva production
- Corneal damage due to poor tear production
- Focal lymphocyte infiltration of the salivary glands
- Studies showing impaired salivary gland function
- Auto-antibody production (Anti-SSA/RO and/or Anti-SSB/LA)

With a positive biopsy or auto-antibodies plus 4/6, the criteria are 97% sensitive and 90% specific for a diagnosis of Sjögren's. Patients with this disorder are at a higher risk for lymphoproliferative complications such as monoclonal gammopathy, type II mixed cryoglobulinemia, non-Hodgkin lymphoma and mucosa-associated lymphoid tissue (MALT).

Board Testing Point: Recognize the association between Sjögren syndrome and NHL.

---

486. Answer: D

Answer: Aerobic, anaerobic, and fungal blood cultures.
This is a case of candidal endophthalmitis associated with fungemia from intravenous methamphetamine abuse. The injected drug suspension frequently includes fungal elements if the lemon juice used to break down the drug rocks becomes contaminated with yeast (candida). Commonly, the pre-squeezed bottles of lemon juice are the most contaminated; yet many patients presume they are sterile and preferentially buy them over lemon fruits. If this patient remains fungemic, as his fever would suggest, routine blood cultures have a sensitivity of nearly 50%. Specific fungal blood cultures will increase the sensitivity slightly. HIV infection can cause a retinopathy, but the appearance is different from that of an endophthalmitis. Excising and culturing the needle and performing a vitrectomy may assist in isolating the fungus, but these procedures are invasive and potentially unnecessary if the organism can be grown in blood cultures. These ocular findings are not consistent with cryptococcal meningitis. Of course, an HIV test should be performed given this patient's drug habit, but the test results will not assist you in diagnosis of his eye condition.

Board Testing Point: Identify the association between lemon juice, methamphetamine, and candida and ocular infections in an IV drug user.

---

487. Answer: B

Answer: Retinal artery occlusion.
A painless loss of vision with a cherry red spot (as shown in the picture) is diagnostic for this condition. All of the other options are painless, except for endophthalmitis. Retinal detachment would show retinal separation. Retinal vein occlusion would show retinal hemorrhage. Occipital cortex infarct would not show any changes in the retina during the immediate post-infarct stage.

Board Testing Point: Recognize the characteristic sign for retinal artery occlusion.

488. Answer: B

Answer: Acyclovir.
Herpes viral infections of the eye are serious conditions and have a high risk for long-term vision compromise. These occur with both herpes simplex and herpes zoster flares. Herpetic lesions on the nose (Hutchinson sign) follow nerve involvement of the nasociliary root. Not all cases of herpetic conjunctivitis demonstrate dendritic (frond-like) lesions but, when present, they are pathognomonic for herpes involvement. Treatment is centered on acyclovir, and the patient usually requires oral or even IV therapy. The nasal lesions may develop impetiginous involvement and benefit from oral antibiotics, but topical ciprofloxacin or erythromycin would not be indicated for the conjunctival component. In very severe cases, topical steroids may be used, but generally they are contraindicated and should not be used without the active involvement of an ophthalmologist.

Board Testing Point: Recognize seriousness of herpes viral infection when it affects the eyes and know treatment.

PSYCHIATRY

489. Answer: B

Answer: Elevated TSH.
Lithium is an effective therapy for bipolar disease and is noted to reduce suicide risk if the levels are maintained (> 0.8 mEq/L). Lithium therapy can reduce urine-concentrating capacity with extended usage, but nephrotoxicity is not a common occurrence. Pancreatitis is a rare side effect with valproic acid therapy, another treatment option for bipolar disorder, but it is not a significant risk with lithium. No Parkinson-like symptoms are described with lithium usage. Lithium does have a significant thyroid effect, interfering with both synthesis and release of thyroid hormone.

Board Testing Point: Know the side effects for lithium.

490. Answer: C

Answer: Keep a sitter at the bedside.
This patient has delirium and has no history of alcohol use. The appropriate initial management should include reversing any modifiable conditions (treat infection, stop offending drugs, etc.) and to work on helping with orientation (keeping the blinds open during the day, clocks, calendars, verbal stimuli). Put her glasses back on if she wears them and return her hearing aids. If she is still agitated, having a sitter available to keep her from getting out of bed is the best option. Restraints will worsen the delirium. Avoid medications if at all possible. Using medication should not be the first-line treatment for delirium.

Board Testing Point: Management of delirium in an ICU patient, especially an elderly patient.

491. Answer: B

Answer: Reduced bone mass.
Most of the physiologic sequelae associated with anorexia nervosa are related to caloric deprivation and improve when body mass approaches therapeutic goals. Menstrual abnormalities, renal abnormalities, and thyroid function normalize in most recovered patients. Obesity is a very uncommon outcome among these patients. Reduced bone mass, however, is a frequent finding. This is felt to arise from impaired gonadal hormones and the effects of increased cortisol levels seen in anorexic patients. The earlier in adolescence that eating disorders begin, the more severe the reduction in bone mass tends to be. Following weight restoration, the reduced bone mass often does not resolve.

Board Testing Point: Loss of bone mass may be permanent in patients with history of anorexia nervosa.

492. Answer: B

Answer: Antidepressants, such as fluoxetine.
Bulimia nervosa (BN) is an eating disorder that involves binges of food intake followed by either purging or periods of food deprivation. Most patients with this condition display few physical findings or laboratory abnormalities, although induced vomiting and laxative and diuretic abuse can produce electrolyte abnormalities. This condition is reported as very uncommon in developing nations, implicating a significant influence from the American culture. There is not a recognized genetic basis at this time. Few patients experience serious

physiological effects and, unlike anorexia nervosa, hospitalization is generally not appropriate. Cognitive behavioral therapy is the initial intervention in many cases. Fluoxetine has also been approved for the treatment of BN.

Board Testing Point: Be familiar with the characteristics of bulimia.

493. Answer: E

Answer: Age of onset.
Attention deficit disorder is a challenging disease to manage due to the subjective nature of the diagnostic criteria and the abuse potential of many of the agents used to control it. Substance abuse is a common co-morbidity in many psychiatric disorders, and the cause/effect interactions are often difficult to distinguish. Presentations of both ADD and BD commonly include substance abuse, emotional lability, poor impulse control, and dysfunctional social interactions. Sleep disturbances are also common to both disorders.

An important criterion for the diagnosis of ADD is demonstration of the disorder before the age of 7 years. This patient's late onset and the absence of dysfunction prior to the age of 13 makes the diagnosis of ADD very suspect and favors an alternative diagnosis, such as BD.

Board Testing Point: Recognize the criteria for attention deficit disorder and bipolar disorder.

494. Answer: E

Answer: Bradycardia.
The toxidrome associated with narcotic overdose consists of decreased level of consciousness, respiratory depression, hypotension, bradycardia, and miosis.

Board Testing Point: Know the signs and symptoms associated with narcotic overdose.

495. Answer: B

Answer: Delayed ejaculation.
The most common cause for discontinuation of SSRIs is sexual side effects. These side effects occur in 30-50% of patients, and the most common sexual side effect is delayed orgasm (ejaculation in men). This side effect is beneficial in men with premature ejaculation, and paroxetine is approved for treatment of this condition.

Board Testing Point: Recognize that most SSRIs have sexual side effects, and that the most common one is delayed ejaculation. On the other hand, SSRIs have been beneficial in treating premature ejaculation.

496. Answer: B

Answer: Tricyclic antidepressants (TCA).
Depression can be a debilitating condition that recurs over spans of years and even decades. Effective medications are increasingly available, and each class of antidepressant has its own side effect profile. The TCA class is noted for its potential to affect cardiac conduction, and prolongation of the QT interval is a serious side effect, particularly in an overdose situation. An individual with known cardiac conduction defects should generally avoid therapy with TCA; close monitoring is recommended, even in patients with no known cardiac compromise.

Board Testing Point: Recognize the association of tricyclic antidepressants and cardiac abnormalities.

497. Answer: D

Answer: Dysthymic disorder.
Dysthymic disorder consists of a persistent, long-term change in mood that generally is less intense but more chronic than occurs in major depressive disorder. The symptoms of dysthymic disorder may not be as severe, but they can cause more psychosocial impairment. For dysthymia to be diagnosed, depressed mood must occur for most of the day, occurring more days than not, and be accompanied by at least 2 of the following:

1. Poor appetite or overeating
2. Insomnia or hypersomnia
3. Low energy or fatigue
4. Low self-esteem
5. Poor concentration
6. Difficulty with making decisions
7. Feelings of hopelessness

This is very difficult to differentiate from major depression, which has to have at least 5 of the following for most of the day, every day, for the past 2 weeks:

1. Depressed mood
2. Loss of interest or pleasure in usual activities
3. Significant weight loss or gain
4. Insomnia or hypersomnia
5. Psychomotor agitation or retardation
6. Fatigue or loss of energy
7. Feelings of worthlessness or excessive or inappropriate guilt
8. Diminished ability to think or concentrate
9. Recurrent thoughts of suicide or death

So it can be difficult to tease out if they try and pin you down on the Boards. A clue for dysthymia is to look for buzzwords like "gloomy outlook on life" or "an underlying sense of inadequacy."

Board Testing Point: Recognize the symptoms of dysthymia.

498. Answer: D

Answer: Panic disorder.
Panic disorder is characterized by the spontaneous and unexpected occurrence of panic attacks. Panic attacks are a period of intense fever in which 4 of 13 defined symptoms develop quickly and peak rapidly less than 10 minutes from onset.

The following symptoms are possible and make up the 13:

1. Palpitations, pounding heart, or accelerated heart rate
2. Sweating
3. Trembling or shaking
4. Sense of shortness of breath or smothering
5. Feeling of choking
6. Chest pain or discomfort
7. Nausea or abdominal distress
8. Feeling dizzy, unsteady, lightheaded, or faint

9. Derealization or depersonalization (feeling detached from oneself)
10. Fear of losing control or going crazy
11. Fear of dying
12. Numbness or tingling sensations
13. Chills or hot flashes

Women outnumber men 2-3-fold; the highest incidence is in late adolescence and then a second peak in the mid-30s. All of the other disorders listed are on the differential, but are MUCH less common.

Board Testing Point: Recognize the signs and symptoms panic disorder.

499. Answer: B

Answer: Agoraphobia.
Agoraphobia is defined as the fear of being alone in a public places (like the supermarket), particularly places where a rapid exit would be difficult in the course of a panic attack. More than 75% of patients with agoraphobia also have panic disorder. Sympathetic nervous system activation is common and results in all of the symptoms that she has. It is more common in women. Most cases occur or begin in adolescence or early adulthood; however, specific triggers (like the fire alarm incident) can trigger the disorder in older individuals.

Board Testing Point: Recognize the signs and symptoms of agoraphobia.

500. Answer: C

Answer: Haloperidol.
He has neuroleptic malignant syndrome, an idiosyncratic response to potent neuroleptics that results in autonomic dysfunction, extrapyramidal symptoms, and high fever. The neuroleptics most commonly involved include haloperidol, piperazine phenothiazines, and thiothixene. Neuroleptic malignant syndrome is thought to be due to depletion of dopamine. It persists for up to 10 days after the drug is stopped. Treatment includes stopping the drug and cooling the patient. Bromocriptine, an oral dopamine agonist, has been shown to be helpful as well.

Board Testing Point: Recognize the neuroleptic malignant syndrome.

501. Answer: D

Answer: Lithium.
She has all of the symptoms of bipolar disorder. Patients with bipolar disorder may never have a depressive episode. Most manic patients are euphoric and have inflated self-esteem, decreased need for sleep, and pressured speech. Hypersexuality is common, as is overspending. Some patients are just irritable. Psychotic symptoms are common during manic episodes. Lithium is effective treatment in 75% of cases, but therapeutic response is very slow (4-6 weeks for full effect) so antipsychotics are often simultaneously started for acute manic episodes. She has no physical signs of hyperthyroidism and other drugs listed would not help with bipolar disorder.

Board Testing Point: Be able to identify bipolar disorder and know its treatment.

502. Answer: D

Answer: Hypophosphatemia.
Many anorexic patients will also purge, thus frequently they have a hypokalemic, hypocalcemic metabolic alkalosis due to the vomiting. Ionized calcium levels usually detect hypocalcemia. Hyponatremia may be seen due to excessive water intake. Low serum phosphorus is common and should be replaced. Interestingly, albumin levels are usually normal. Thyroid function tests are generally normal.

Board Testing Point: Recognize the electrolyte abnormalities associated with anorexia nervosa.

503. Answer: C

Answer: Discuss with him the need for hospitalization and ask him for voluntary admission; if he refuses, then institute emergency commitment.
This patient has definite suicidal ideation and has a plan, as recently as the morning of his appointment. Although he says he is not suicidal in your office, the recent events suggest that he is not stable and requires immediate hospitalization for his own protection. It is always best to try and initiate voluntary admission, which many patients will adhere to; but if he refuses, then emergency commitment is warranted. It is not appropriate to have anything but inpatient admission at this point.

Board Testing Point: Recognize the need for immediate hospitalization in the case of significant suicidal ideation or attempt.

504. Answer: A

Answer: Enlarged right atrium.
Lithium use during pregnancy is associated with Ebstein anomaly. Findings include downward displacement of the tricuspid valve into the right ventricle. The anterior cusp of the valve is partially attached to the valve ring, but other leaflets are adherent to the wall of the ventricle. The right ventricle is therefore divided into two parts creating a huge right atrium and small inefficient right ventricle. Symptoms vary from mild (fatigue, palpitations) to severe (cyanosis and cardiomegaly), depending on degree of displacement of the tricuspid valve and the severity of the obstruction to the right ventricular outflow tract.

Board Testing Point: Recognize that lithium use during pregnancy is associated with Ebstein anomaly.

505. Answer: B

Answer: Hypokalemia.
The patient presents with several symptoms consistent with bulimia. The parotid gland often is enlarged as a result of self induced vomiting. Soft palate petechiae represent injury from fingers scratching the palate during attempts to induce vomiting; the fingers often show bruises or calluses over the knuckles. Hypokalemia is often associated with a decrease in chloride on metabolic screening, i.e., hypochloremic, hypokalemic metabolic alkalosis. Serious cardiac arrhythmias may result in syncope or sudden cardiac death.

Board Testing Point: Diagnose bulimia based on physical examination and predict the laboratory abnormalities associated with chronic purging.

506. Answer: D

Answer: Abnormal sex chromosome karyotype results
He has Klinefelter Syndrome, the most common sex chromosome aneuploidy in males. This question was placed in the psychiatry section because many of these individuals are evaluated for social disorders or "difficulty relating" to peers, and come in more for psychological complaints than physical. The Boards know this and may try to make you think he just has psychological issues and veil the physical findings deep in the question.

Most patients have a 47, XXY complement on chromosome testing although some have mosaic patterns. Gonadotropin levels are not elevated until mid puberty when testicular growth usually stops, resulting in infertility in the vast majority of patients. Testosterone levels are slightly low, and replacement therapy with a long-acting testosterone is usually recommended starting at 11-12 years of age. Polycystic kidney disease is not associated with Klinefelter Syndrome.

Board Testing Point: Recognize that psychological issues may be the primary complaint in an adolescent or young adult with underlying physical disorder.

507. Answer: D

Answer: Ceruloplasmin level.
The patient has Wilson disease, or hepatolenticular degeneration, due to defective mobilization of copper from lysosomes for excretion into the bile. Copper accumulates in the liver; when retention capacity is exceeded, the copper escapes and accumulates in the brain, kidney and cornea. Liver abnormalities include hepatomegaly, hepatitis, cirrhosis, portal hypertension and hepatic failure. Neuropsychiatric disorders include behavioral changes, decrease in school performance, tremors, dysarthria, and dystonia. Copper accumulation in the cornea leads to the formation of concentric rings known as Kayser-Fleischer rings. Decreased ceruloplasmin level, elevated serum copper, and elevated urinary excretion of copper are diagnostic.

Treatment with penicillamine leads to improvement. Foods high in copper, including liver, shellfish, nuts, and chocolate, should be avoided. Maternal blood alpha-fetoprotein levels (AFP) are used as a screening test for Trisomy 21, and some hepatomas and germ cell tumors also secrete AFP in abnormal amounts; haptoglobin binds free hemoglobin and is decreased in hemolytic anemias; total iron binding capacity is increased in iron deficiency anemia; free erythrocyte protoporphyrin is elevated in lead poisoning and iron deficiency anemia.

Board Testing Point: Recognize that Wilson disease frequently presents with psychiatric abnormalities before gastrointestinal signs/symptoms occur.

508. Answer: A

Answer: Gynecomastia.
Several drugs of abuse, including marijuana (cannabis), heroin, methadone, and amphetamines, may cause gynecomastia. Other drugs associated with this clinical finding include phenothiazines, spironolactone, cimetidine, isoniazid, ketoconazole, estrogen and anabolic steroids. Marijuana use may lead to hypertension and tachycardia as well as elevated temperature. Patients may also report symptoms of pharyngitis, sinusitis and asthma, especially with chronic use.

Board Testing Point: Recognize the potential sequelae from long-term use of illicit drugs.

MISCELLANEOUS

509. Answer: C

Answer: 57%.

An easy way to determine the operating characteristics of a diagnostic test given the prevalence of disease, sensitivity / specificity of the test, and percent of abnormal results (or other combinations of operating characteristics) is to use a 2 x 2 table, shown below. Recall that sensitivity is often referred to as "positive in disease," and is the number of true positive tests divided by the total number of patients with the disease (TP/TP+FN). Specificity, known by the phrase "negative in health," is the number of normal tests found in all patients who do not have the disease (TN/TN+FP). Positive predictive value is the number of accurate positive tests out of all positive tests (TP/TP+FP); negative predictive value is the number of accurate normal tests out of all patients whose test is normal (TN/TN+FN). Prevalence of disease may have dramatic effects on the PPV and NPV of a test (testing for a disease with low prevalence, even if the test is highly sensitive, will have a lower PPV than testing for a disease with a higher prevalence).

In our example, the 2 x 2 box would look like this (assuming a population of 100,000):

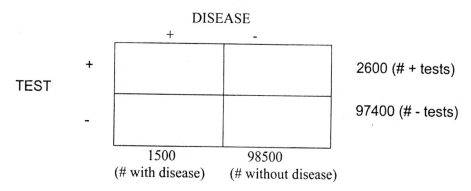

Then, knowing the test is 98% sensitive, the top left box may be filled in (98% of 1500 patients with disease = 1470), followed by simple subtraction for the rest of the box:

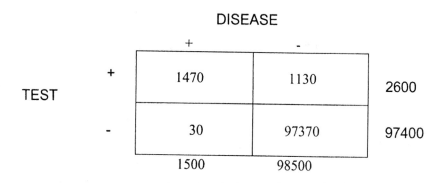

Then, to calculate the positive predictive value: 1470 / (1470+1130) = **56.5%**.

As an example of the effect of prevalence on PPV, look at the calculation of PPV if the disease prevalence is only 1/250 (0.4%):

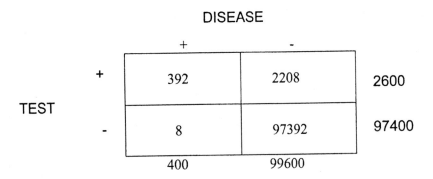

Giving a PPV of 392/ (392+2208) = **15%.**

Board Testing Point: To understand sensitivity/specificity/other operating characteristics of diagnostic tests.

---

510. Answer: D

Answer: Grapefruit juice.
Grapefruit juice has an effect on the CY3A subunit of the P450 system and decreases metabolism of nifedipine. Nifedipine doses should be separated from grapefruit juice intake by at least an hour. Grapefruit juice also markedly increases the concentration of statins such as lovastatin and simvastatin. The other beverages listed do not affect nifedipine or statins.

Board Testing Point: Interpret the interactions between medications and grapefruit juice

---

511. Answer: A

Answer: There is no statistically significant evidence of protection from breastfeeding.
For all of the studies, the 95% confidence intervals cross 1, meaning that there is greater than 5% chance the results are due to chance (P of < .05 is considered statistically significant). For odds ratios (OR), you would look for the 95% CI to span below 1. For example, a "statistically significant" study would be an odds ratio of 0.6 with a 95% CI of 0.45 to 0.7. With an OR of 0.6 and a significant CI, this study would demonstrate that breastfeeding does reduce the risk of breast cancer.

Board Testing Point: Interpret odds ratios (OR) and confidence intervals (CI)

---

512. Answer: B

Answer: A dosage error was made, and he received 10x the insulin dose he was supposed to receive; therefore, he is receiving a glucose infusion to help prevent low blood sugar.
It is appropriate to disclose this error fully. Tell him he received 10x the appropriate dose of insulin. Also tell him what steps are being done to prevent problems related to this error. It is never appropriate to "hide" or withhold this type of information from the patient. It is also not ethical to discuss the incident only if the patient initiates the conversation. Physicians should be open with all errors.

Board Testing Point: Ethics: notification of physician/hospital errors.

513. Answer: D

Answer: Blood glucose monitoring is not associated with a statistically significant change in HbA1C.
The correct answer is that there is no statistically significant evidence that blood glucose monitoring leads to lower hemoglobin A1C levels. All of the confidence intervals cross zero, which indicates that the studies are not significant. Also, the "combined" analysis reveals the same finding. To be statistically significant, the values must be either above 0 or below 0. Example: If one of the studies has a mean value of -1.5 with a 95% CI (-1.3 to -1.7), this would be statistically significant.

Board Testing Point: Interpretation of 95% confidence intervals

514. Answer: E

Answer: Cleansing of the canal and biopsy of granulation tissue.
Malignant otitis externa is an invasive process that originates in the external ear canal and can slowly erode through surrounding bony structures, potentially leading to osteomyelitis and meningitis. Immune compromise, diabetes mellitus, and advanced age are risk factors for developing malignant otitis externa. This condition resembles chronic otitis externa with swelling and erythema of the ear canal, often with purulent discharge. However, malignant otitis externa develops granulation tissue, typically in the posterior inferior wall of the canal, which serves as the infection nidus and results in the erosive process.

Pseudomonas is implicated in many cases, but *S. aureus, Actinomyces, Aspergillus,* and some Gram-negative bacteria have also been implicated. Appropriate treatment choices depend on identification of offending organisms through bacterial and fungal cultures. In the absence of osteomyelitis, antimicrobial therapy alone is often curative if the appropriate drugs are selected based on culture results. Surface cultures often reveal multiple organisms that colonize the canal but are not involved in the deeper infection. Cleansing of the canal followed by biopsy of the granulation tissue is most effective in establishing the infecting organisms and their antimicrobial susceptibilities.

Board Testing Point: Manage the diabetic patient with malignant otitis externa.

515. Answer: D

Answer: *Treponema pallidum.*
She has neurosyphilis. The rash she described was likely secondary syphilis. Rubella and rubeola do not commonly cause hearing loss in adults; however, rubella causes significant congenital hearing loss. Lyme disease could potentially cause hearing loss, but it is less common in this geographic location; and the rash described is inconsistent with Lyme disease. Parvovirus B-19 would not cause isolated hearing loss. A 25-year-old will not have early pre-senile hearing loss.

Board Testing Point: Hearing loss in a sexually active young person should raise the suspicion of syphilis.

516. Answer: B

Answer: Cerumen impaction.
There are 2 general categories of hearing loss: 1) sensorineural and 2) conductive. For sensorineural hearing loss to occur, the pathologic process must affect the inner ear, 8th cranial nerve, or the auditory area of the brain. Common causes of sensorineural hearing loss include presbycusis (natural aging), infections, vascular

abnormalities, trauma, tumors, and medications. For a conductive hearing loss to occur, the pathologic process must involve "blocking" the auditory vibrations from reaching the inner ear. Common causes include external canal obstruction (cerumen), otitis externa and media, cholesteatoma, otosclerosis, trauma, and middle ear masses.

Tests to consider when a patient presents with a hearing loss include the Weber and Rinne tests for screening, then audiometry if abnormal. A CT scan should be performed, especially if there is a history of trauma or an MRI if asymmetric sensorineural hearing loss has occurred.

What are those Rinne and Weber tests that you learned in physical diagnosis? The Rinne test helps evaluate for conductive hearing loss, i.e., anything that decreases the amount of sound that gets to the inner ear. In this test a 256 Hz (or 512 Hz) tuning fork is held with the base touching the mastoid process to see how well the sound transmits through the bone to the inner ear. The tuning fork is then held with the tines over the external ear on the same side, and the sounds (tuning fork on the mastoid vs. tuning fork by the external ear) are compared. In normal exams, the air-conducted (i.e., the patient hears better with the tuning fork by the external ear canal than on the mastoid) sounds are louder. If the sound transmitted by bone is louder, the patient has a conduction defect (something either in the external ear or the middle ear is blocking the sound vibrations from reaching the inner ear.) If the patient had sensorineural hearing loss, then all sounds will seem decreased, but the air-conducted sound would still be louder than the bone-conducted sound.

For the Weber test, the tuning fork is held with the base on the mid-forehead. In a normal exam, the sound is perceived in the middle, but this could also be seen in BILATERAL sensorineural hearing loss. If the sound lateralizes to one side (the patient hears it better on one side than the other), it means there is either a conductive hearing loss on the SAME side or a sensorineural hearing loss on the OTHER side.

So, for our patient in this question, the Rinne test heard air conduction better on the left side (normal) and bone conduction was louder on the right side (indicating obstruction of air flow on the right). The Weber test lateralized to the right ear, meaning he either has a conduction defect on the right side or he has a sensorineural hearing loss on the left side. Our Rinne test did not show bilateral sensorineural hearing loss and in fact showed obstruction on the right side as well. Therefore, the most likely etiology of those listed is cerumen impaction on the right.

Gentamicin and Ménière's disease would cause sensorineural hearing loss. Acoustic neuroma and Cochlear osteosclerosis would both cause conductive hearing loss but are MUCH less common than cerumen impaction.

Board Testing Point: Understand how to use the Rinne and Weber tests in determining the etiology of hearing loss.

517. Answer: C

Answer: Vascular disease.
The erectile dysfunction in this 75-year-old man is most likely due to vascular disease. Vascular disease is the 2nd most common cause of erectile dysfunction (diabetes is #1). He has a history of hypertension and coronary artery disease, suggesting that underlying vascular disease is likely. Neuropathy rarely occurs without diabetes. It is unlikely that, at the age of 75, he has a lower testosterone level than he did a few years ago. He has been on the atenolol for years, and it is very unlikely to suddenly cause a problem.

Board Testing Point: Recognize that vascular disease is a common cause of erectile dysfunction in older men.

518. Answer: E

Answer: Sensorineural hearing loss of the left ear.
First let's review the Rinne and Weber tests. The Rinne test helps evaluate for conductive hearing loss, i.e., anything that decreases the amount of sound that gets to the inner ear. In this test a 256 Hz (or 512 Hz) tuning fork is held with the base touching the mastoid process to see how well the sound transmits through the bone to the inner ear. The tuning fork is then held with the tines over the external ear on the same side, and the sounds (tuning fork on the mastoid vs. tuning fork by the external ear) are compared. In normal exams, the air-conducted sounds are louder (i.e.. The patient hears better with the tuning fork by the external ear canal than on the mastoid). If the sound transmitted by bone is louder, the patient has a conduction defect (something either in the external ear or the middle ear is blocking the sound vibrations from reaching the inner ear.) If the patient had sensorineural hearing loss, then all sounds will seem decreased but the air-conducted sound would still be louder than the bone conducted sound.

For the Weber test, the tuning fork is held with the base on the mid-forehead. In a normal exam, the sound is perceived in the middle, but this could also be seen in BILATERAL sensorineural hearing loss. If the sound lateralizes to one side (the patient hears it better on one side than the other), it means there is either a conductive hearing loss on the SAME side or a sensorineural hearing loss on the OTHER side.

So to review the findings of our patient's Rinne and Weber tests: The Weber test is showing that he has either a left sensorineural hearing loss or a conduction abnormality on the right side. The Rinne testing shows that he does not have an obstruction in his right ear. The Rinne tests "rules out" most obstructive causes such as those listed: left TM perforation, acute otitis media, otosclerosis, and excessive cerumen. The only thing that fits his testing scenario is a left-sided sensorineural hearing loss.

Board Testing Point: Interpret the Rinne and Weber tests to determine the etiology of hearing loss.

519. Answer: C

Answer: Argatroban® should be substituted for subcutaneous heparin in the future.
Heparin-induced platelet dysfunction can be mediated by direct agglutination of platelets or by an immune complex reaction. Readministration of unfractionated heparin, even in small amounts, can restimulate the process. Enoxaparin has 10-20% cross-reactivity with pre-existing antibodies to unfractionated heparin. Platelets are the targets of both types of reactions, and platelet infusions are not an effective countermeasure. Argatroban is the current treatment choice in these patients.

Board Testing Point: Recognize "white clot syndrome" and how to effectively anticoagulate a patient with history of this syndrome.

520. Answer: C

Answer: Sweat chloride testing and/or more specific testing for a genetic mutation.
With the finding of *Pseudomonas aeruginosa* in a patient with recurrent sinusitis and possible recurrent bronchitis and pneumonia, the suspicion of cystic fibrosis (CF) should be raised. Unfortunately, an increasing number of cases are being diagnosed in young adults and even in people in their late 20s and 30s. With over 1000 mutations for CF, the phenotypic presentation is variable. The finding of the nasal polyp is nearly pathognomonic in a young person for CF. She is not a candidate for sinus surgery, and repeating the sinus culture is not going to be helpful, particularly if you treat her with ceftriaxone, which does not have anti-pseudomonal coverage. Serum IgE levels would be useful in the diagnosis of Job syndrome, but Job's presents with recurrent *Staphylococcus* infections,

not pseudomonal infections. A nasal smear for eosinophils would be useful if you were suspecting an allergic component, unlikely in this case scenario.

Board Testing Point: Recognize the findings of cystic fibrosis in an undiagnosed young adult.

521. Answer: D

Answer: Testicular ultrasound.
The differential diagnosis of acute scrotal pain includes epididymitis, orchitis, inguinal hernia, and testicular torsion, as well as referred pain from renal stone. Of all of these diagnoses, testicular torsion requires the most immediate attention since delays can lead to testicular loss. The most urgent intervention is to assess for testicular perfusion and, if needed, to reestablish testicular blood flow. Cultures, antibiotic therapy and other interventions can be pursued once the possibility of testicular torsion has been excluded.

Board Testing Point: Evaluate testicular pain in the setting of possible testicular torsion.

522. Answer: A

Answer: HIV infection.
Methamphetamine is a physically addictive drug that is increasing in use across the U.S. As a crystalline powder, it is commonly inhaled nasally but can also be abused through oral, rectal, and IV routes or by smoking. Serious side effects include hyperthermia, rhabdomyolysis, seizures, and stroke. It can also lead to hypertension, tachycardia, palpitations and dysrhythmias. Long-term abusers often experience erectile dysfunction and delayed ejaculation, but priapism is not a common result. Common effects of methamphetamine abuse include increased libido, decreased inhibition, and ulcerations of mucous membranes. This combination has lead to an increased frequency of sexually transmitted diseases, including hepatitis and HIV infection.

Board Testing Point: Associate HIV infection with methamphetamine (crystal meth) use.

523. Answer: E

Answer: Discuss the use of transdermal nicotine patches with the patient.
Patients with long-term usage of nicotine products are subject to significant withdrawal when they are hospitalized without smoking privileges. The distress that accompanies the withdrawal frequently results in patients making decisions that may not be in their best long-term interest. This patient has demonstrated no evidence of psychotic behavior; so a psychiatry consult and the use of antipsychotic medications are not appropriate. Restraining this patient under these circumstances would be both medically and legally irresponsible. The patient does have the right to leave the hospital at her discretion. Before this option is exercised, it would be wise to discuss the use of a nicotine patch to reduce her tobacco-withdrawal symptoms and allow her to complete in-hospital treatment. It may also serve to start a long-term intervention for smoking cessation.

Board Testing Point: Recommend treatment to ameliorate nicotine withdrawal in a long-time smoker.

524. Answer: C

Answer: Have her discuss the issue with your risk management administrator.
The patient is coming to you for assistance. It is not appropriate to refer her to an attorney since you did not witness the alleged actions and, at this point, have been unable to ascertain if the allegations are true. You are

obliged, however, to refer her to someone who can do an independent investigation, and that person would be your risk management administrator. You should talk to your partner and find out if this behavior is a concern, but you should NOT have your partner meet with her. Also, she is a patient of your group, and you cannot "abandon" her and refuse to see her for medical conditions without making appropriate arrangements first; she is NOT responsible for a referral. Until an independent investigation has been completed, it is inappropriate to notify the local medical board. The key is to put the patient in contact with someone who can do a fair, independent investigation.

Board Testing Point: Manage an alleged case of sexual or physical misconduct in the office practice setting.

525. Answer: D

Answer: Discontinue the tube feedings, since this is what the patient has informed you as her wishes. These ethical questions are difficult for many. However, it is quite clear in this instance that the patient has expressed her wishes to you, and you have documented them in her chart. She trusts you to follow her wishes in the face of others wanting something different. It is very clear when a patient's wishes are documented that they should be carried out. Thus it is not appropriate to give her tube feedings at this time, and an ethics consult is unnecessary when patient's wishes are documented clearly. If the daughters want to intervene, they can try court action. But the law is very clear about protecting rights of the individual who has expressed her wishes before becoming incapacitated.

Board Testing Point: Recognize that the documented wishes of a patient outweigh those of the family members, even for those "next-in-line" for making decisions.

526. Answer: D

Answer: Prolonged QT interval.
About 50% of cases of Long QT Syndrome (LQTS) are familial and are frequently due to Romano-Ward Syndrome (autosomal dominant) and Jervell-Lange-Nielsen Syndrome (autosomal recessive and associated with congenital deafness). The remainder of LQTS cases are sporadic. Syncopal episodes associated with LQTS are usually associated with exercise or a sudden frightening event. A heart rate corrected QT interval of > 0.47 seconds is highly correlated with LQTS. Beta-blockers are the initial treatment of choice.

Wenckebach 2nd degree AV block is associated with a PR interval that increases progressively until a P wave is not conducted; Wenckebach is not associated with syncope or progression to heart block. Delta waves are associated with Wolff-Parkinson-White Syndrome, and syncope associated with WPW occurs during times of tachycardia. A wandering atrial pacemaker is defined by a shift in the pacemaker of the heart from the sinus node to another part of the atrium. ST segment depression is indicative of hypoxic injury to cardiac tissue.

Board Testing Point: Associate genetic deafness due to Jervell-Lange-Nielsen Syndrome with Long QT Syndrome.

527. Answer: B

Answer: Increased width of the retropharyngeal space with an air-fluid level on lateral roentgenogram.
He has a retropharyngeal abscess as a result of a penetrating injury to the soft palate caused by the stick in his mouth. Such an injury results in the introduction of organisms residing in the oropharynx into the retropharyngeal space. Patients with a retropharyngeal abscess often hold their necks in a hyperextended position, as compared to those with epiglottitis, who often sit leaning forward. Retropharyngeal abscesses used to be exclusively a disease

of children but are now increasingly seen in adults; a review from Brooklyn NY showed that 70% occurred in adults aged 21-64 years. Emergent consultation with an ENT specialist is necessary. "Asymmetric tonsillar bulge with deviation of the uvula on examination of the oropharynx" describes a peritonsillar abscess; although patients with this disorder may present in a similar fashion, a history of falling with an object in the mouth is characteristic of an abscess in the retropharyngeal space. The clinical findings are not consistent with a displaced tooth or foreign body.

Board Testing Point: Recognize the findings of a retropharyngeal abscess and that its incidence is increasing in adults.

---

528. Answer: C

Answer: Nasal foreign body.
The presence of a nasal foreign body often acts as an irritant leading to mucosal edema, partial nasal obstruction and infection associated with a malodorous, often unilateral, discharge which may also be bloody. Although the vignette also describes signs of allergy ("allergic shiners," dark red purple circles beneath the eyes), a unilateral foul smelling discharge is typical of a nasal foreign body. Chronic sinusitis may be associated with malodorous breath but not unilateral discharge. Cough variant asthma would be very unusual in this patient, and a nasal polyp would not cause these symptoms.

Board Testing Point: Diagnose nasal foreign body by assessment of history and physical examination, noticing unilateral drainage.

---

529. Answer: D

Answer: Waning immunity among adolescents and adults has resulted in an increase in the number of cases of pertussis in this population, leading to transmission of disease to unimmunized and under-immunized populations.
Over the last several decades, the number of reported cases of pertussis has continued to increase. In large part this is a result of waning immunity in adolescents and adults. Although disease is milder in older individuals, they serve as reservoirs of infection, transmitting the organism to infants and toddlers at highest risk of morbidity and mortality. These circumstances have led to the recent recommendation to immunize adolescents AND adults (19-64 years of age) with one Tdap vaccine to provide a pertussis booster as well as tetanus and diphtheria. The new Tdap replaces the Td booster in adults.

Board Testing Point: Recognize that pertussis is becoming more common in adults, and vaccination of all adults ages 19-64 with one Tdap booster instead of Td is recommended.

---

530. Answer: C

Answer: The catarrhal stage of pertussis is difficult to clinically distinguish from an otherwise uncomplicated upper respiratory infection.
After an incubation phase of 1-2 weeks, pertussis disease has three phases: catarrhal, paroxysmal, and convalescent. The catarrhal stage presents as a typical, uncomplicated upper respiratory infection lasting between 5-12 days. During the catarrhal stage, patients are most infectious. It is not until the paroxysmal stage develops, with its characteristic paroxysms of coughing followed by a "whoop," that pertussis becomes clinically apparent. After 1-2 weeks, this stage is followed by an often prolonged (several weeks-months) convalescent stage. Patients with pertussis often have a prominent lymphocytosis associated with an elevated WBC count. Adolescents and adults, despite being fully immunized earlier in life, often develop pertussis due to waning vaccine immunity.

COLOR SLIDES

Question 79

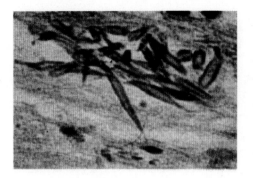

Question 186

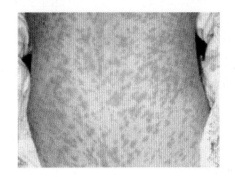

Question 108

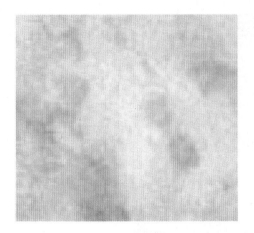

Question 187

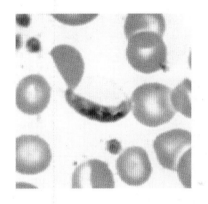

Question 179

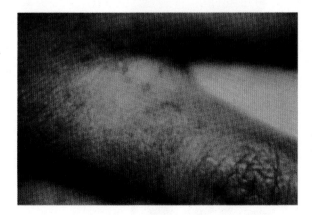

Question 192

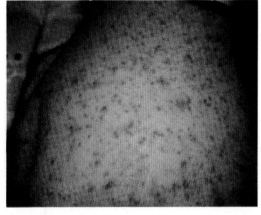

COLOR SLIDES

Question 193

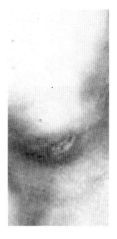

Question 201

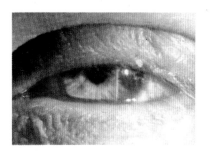

Question 203

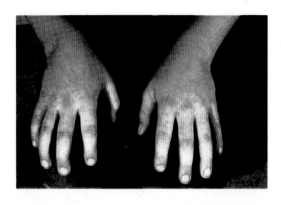

Question 204

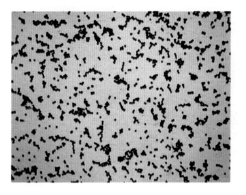

Question 211

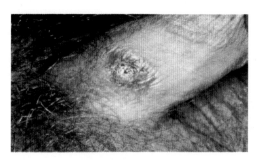

Question 213

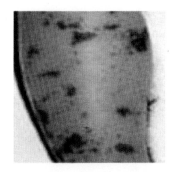

Question 216

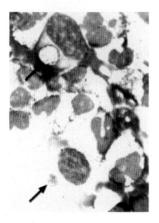

COLOR SLIDES

Question 219

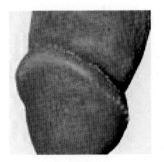

Question 221

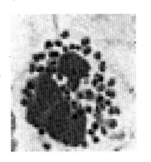

Question 226

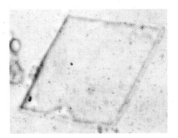

Question 232

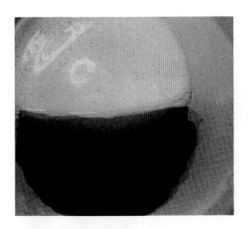

Question 261

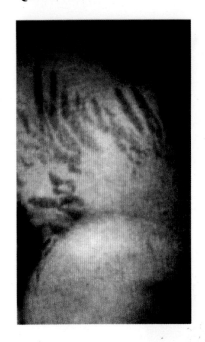

Question 266

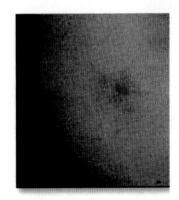

Question 267

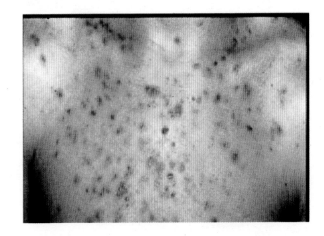

COLOR SLIDES

Question 270

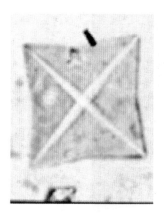

Question 319

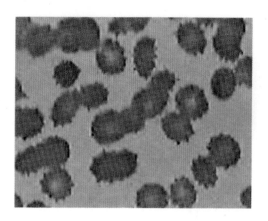

Question 273

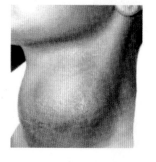

Question 320

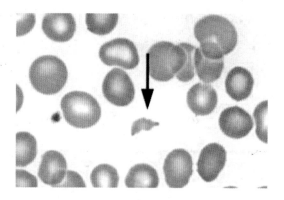

Question 317

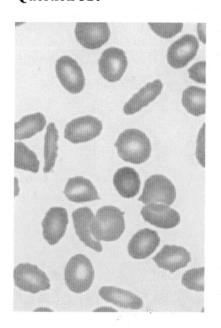

Question 321

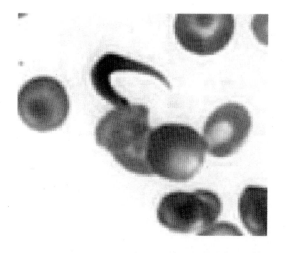

Question 318

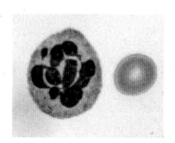

COLOR SLIDES

Question 322

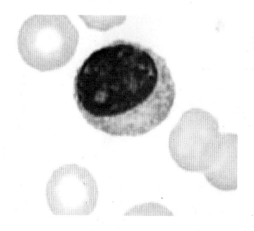

Question 325

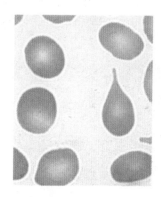

Question 323

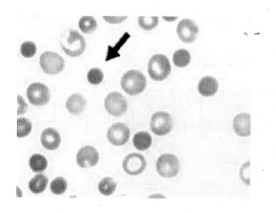

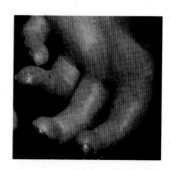

Question 352

Question 324

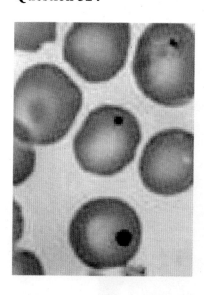

Question 393

COLOR SLIDES

Question 400

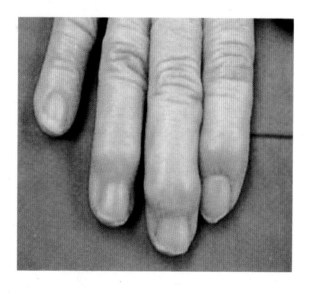

Question 444

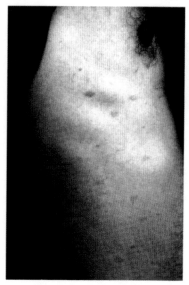

Question 442

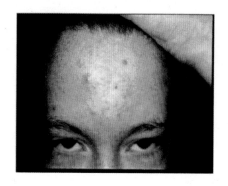

Question 445

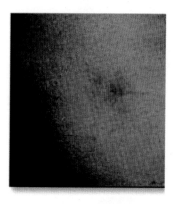

Question 443

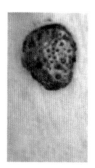

Question 446

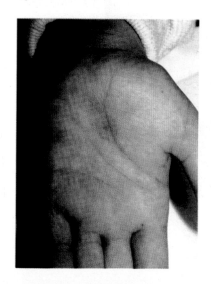

COLOR SLIDES

Question 447

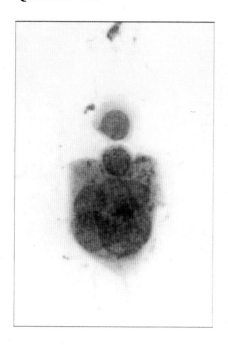

Question 454

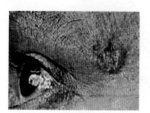

Question 455

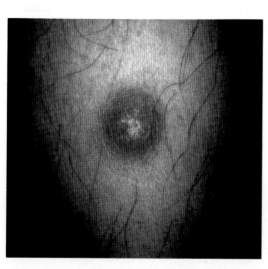

Question 457

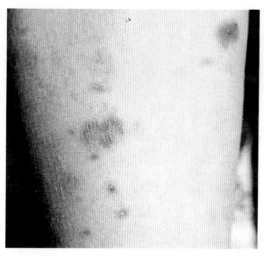

Question 458

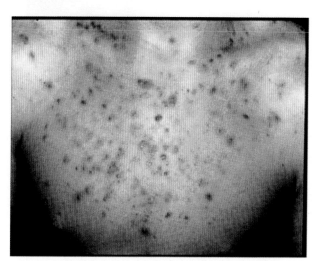

Question 459

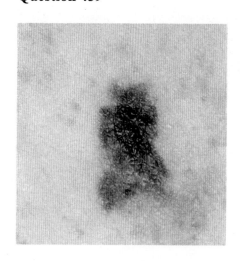

COLOR SLIDES

Question 460

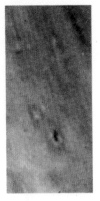

Question 461

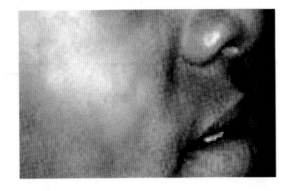

Question 480

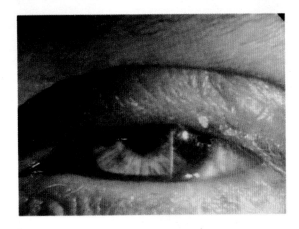

Question 487

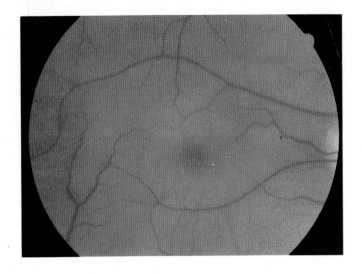

Question 507

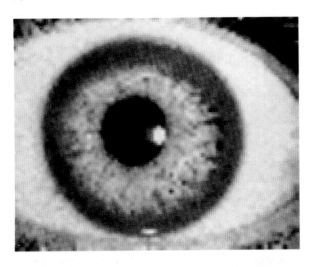